INFECTIOUS CHANGE

KATHERINE A. MASON

Infectious Change

Reinventing Chinese Public Health
After an Epidemic

Stanford University Press · *Stanford, California*

Stanford University Press
Stanford, California

Printed in the United States of America on acid-free, archival-quality paper

Library of Congress Cataloging-in-Publication Data
Names: Mason, Katherine A. (Katherine Anne), author.
Title: Infectious change : reinventing Chinese public health after an
    epidemic / Katherine A. Mason.
Description: Stanford, California : Stanford University Press, 2016. |
    Includes bibliographical references and index.
Identifiers: LCCN 2015050118 | ISBN 9780804794435 (cloth : alk. paper) |
    ISBN 9780804798921 (pbk. : alk. paper) | ISBN 9780804798952 (ebook)
Subjects: LCSH: Public health—China, Southeast. | Public health
    administration—China, Southeast. | SARS (Disease)—China,
    Southeast.
Classification: LCC RA395.C6 M37 2016 | DDC 362.10951—dc23
LC record available at http://lccn.loc.gov/2015050118

Typeset by Thompson Type in 9.75/13.5 Janson

For my family: past, present, and future

Contents

Acknowledgments

Like so many scholars, I must begin this book with a statement of apology about the impossibility of adequately thanking all of the people who made my work possible. The debts of gratitude that I owe to my informants, colleagues, family members, and mentors are innumerable and immeasurable, and I am sure I will never be able to sufficiently thank all those who should be thanked. And yet I must try my best.

First and foremost, I extend my deep and heartfelt gratitude to all those at the Tianmai CDC and elsewhere in Tianmai, Guangzhou, Beijing, and Hong Kong who opened their lives to me and shared so much and so generously. Though I am not able to list their real names here, I hope that they know how grateful I am to all of them for their willingness to welcome a foreigner into their world and to trust me with their stories. Their friendship means the world to me. In particular, I am deeply grateful to the man I call Director Lan, who made it possible for me to work at the TM CDC; Lan's wife, a dear friend who remains unnamed in the text but whose ideas and passions resonate throughout; Lan's assistant, who became my protector and roommate and who also remains unnamed but appears in various key places in the text; and the woman I call Xu Dan, whose friendship, openness, and insights drove many of the analyses in this work. I hope that these and my dozens of other interlocutors understand that whatever critiques and suggestions I raise in these pages are offered with respect and affection and with the hope that bringing such issues to light might in some way help them to find whatever it is they are looking for. I also ask for their forgiveness if my necessary but clumsy efforts to conceal their identities and the identity of Tianmai fail to prevent them from receiving unwanted attention from the wrong places.

This book is the product of a search for meaning that began on the day I was evacuated from Guangzhou during the SARS epidemic in April 2003. I never would have gone to China in the first place, let alone had that life-changing experience, without the opportunities afforded to me by the Yale-China Association. I thank all of the folks who made Yale-China so great during my 2001–2003 tenure as a Teaching Fellow, especially Julia Travers, Andy Junker, and Nancy Chapman. I also thank my fellow Yale-China fellows, many of whom became lifelong friends and colleagues, including Sarah Donaldson, Denise Ho, Aaron Lichtig, Hari Osofsky, and Margaret Boittin.

Special thanks go to three other wonderful women whom I met in my early days in Guangzhou. I first met Wang Jing and Chen Wei in 2001, when they were students in my English class at Zhongshan University in Guangzhou. They taught me a great deal of important slang and fed me a great deal of delicious food, and I am deeply grateful for their ongoing friendship and support. Wang Jing has welcomed me into her home countless times over the past fourteen years and always had a bed and a bowl of dumplings ready for me whenever I went to Guangzhou during my fieldwork. She also checked over most of the translations in the book and is now an anthropologist in her own right. I owe her a great deal. Chen Wei provided me with a home and many delicious meals during my return trips to China in 2010 and 2014. She also spent much of her free time in 2008 and 2009 expertly transcribing almost all of the nearly 100 taped Chinese-language interviews that provided much of the ethnographic material for this book. Her insights also were extremely helpful to me in thinking through my analysis. I am deeply grateful to her as well. Finally, Xie Jianmei has for nearly a decade been friend, language partner, and colleague and has provided informal research assistance at several points along the way. In Guangzhou I also thank Lynn Cai, Feng Yichong ("Lao Zhongyi"), Zhou Daming, Cheng Yu, and myriad unnamed informants who appear in these pages. In Hong Kong I am especially grateful to Joseph Lau.

Research for this book was conducted with the generous support of the Social Science Research Council, Wenner-Gren Foundation, Fulbright-IIE, and Association for Asian Studies. Funds for follow-up research in 2014 and for the indexing of this book were provided by the Robert Wood Johnson Foundation Health and Society Scholars program. Support for research assistance in preparing the final manuscript were provided by the Brown University Population Studies and Training Center. I am grateful to have had the privilege of so much generous research support.

I am also very thankful to have been a part of many wonderful communities of scholars who have at various points along this long road spurred me to think more deeply and more broadly about my work. From my Harvard days I thank Priscilla Song, Sarah Willen, Zhang Min, Vanessa Fong, Maria Stalford, Jesse Grayman, Denise Ho, Emilio Dirlikov, and Sharon Abramowitz. Special thanks go to Elanah Uretsky for reading and offering careful critiques of several chapter drafts, and to Nicole Newendorp and Rubie Watson for providing key insights on early versions of Chapter One. A special shout-out goes to Felicity Aulino, who has read iterations of certain chapters in this book more times than I can count and has also provided many years of moral support. My fieldwork time in Tianmai was greatly enhanced by the intellectual companionship of Mary Ann O'Donnell, Winnie Wong, Margaret Boittin, and Miguel De Figueiredo. While at Harvard I also benefited from the feedback and insights of Andrew Kipnis and Susan Greenhalgh.

Some of my deepest debts of gratitude go to my graduate mentors at Harvard. James "Woody" Watson was relentless in his encouragement and in his nagging to "keep my eye on the ball." Duana Fullwiley provided detailed and incisive feedback that was always extremely productive. I am grateful to Charles Rosenberg for his timely feedback, his willingness to be frank and direct, his valuable historical perspective, and his overall good humor. Finally, I owe an immeasurable debt of gratitude to my primary advisor, Arthur Kleinman, whose unbending support of me and unflagging belief in the worth of this project drove me forward. Arthur's brilliance, his uncanny ability to identify and articulate exactly what I was trying to say long before I realized I wanted to say it, and his unflagging dedication and loyalty to his students, his family, and his life's work continue to inspire me.

At the University of Pennsylvania Department of History and Sociology of Science I was privileged to work with many wonderful scholars and students who took me out of my comfort zone and made me think more historically and globally. I thank all of my students in the Health and Societies program at Penn, as well as my colleagues in the department, including David Barnes, Robert Aronowitz, Ruth Cowan, and Patricia Johnson. At Penn, Beth Linker, Lisa Messeri, and Jessica Mozersky deserve special mention for their ongoing scholarly feedback and their friendship.

The Robert Wood Johnson Foundation Health and Society Scholars program at Columbia University (2013–2015) provided the time, space, and funds to do much of the writing and rewriting of this book. It also provided an interdisciplinary intellectual environment that proved especially fruitful for rethinking the manuscript at critical stages. My year of residency at the Mailman School of Public Health as a RWJF HSS scholar between 2013 and 2014 was invaluable in helping me to understand public health from not just a Chinese perspective but an American one as well. At Columbia I thank Peter Bearman, Julien Teitler, Kathy Neckerman, Lisa Bates, Valerie Purdie-Vaughn, Adam Reich, Chris Muller, Jon Zelner, Elizabeth Wrigley-Field, Michael Falco, and DiLenny Roca-Dominguez. Special thanks go to Bruce Link for his mentorship and encouragement, Sarah Cowan and Natalie Brito for their companionship and commiseration, and Larry Yang for his collaborative spirit. Special thanks also go to Sammy Zahran, who in reading the first few pages of a draft of my introduction in the fall of 2013 produced a critical insight that helped me to frame the entire book.

Since arriving at Brown University in the fall of 2014, I have been privileged to join a warm and collegial intellectual community in the Department of Anthropology and beyond. I thank my colleagues in the Department and at the Population Studies and Training Center for their support and for their feedback on various portions of this work, including Daniel Smith, Andrew Foster, Jessaca Leinaweaver, David Kertzer, Bhrigupati Singh, Rebecca Carter, Sherine Hamdy, Paja Faudree, Adia Benton, Matthew Gutmann, Catherine Lutz, William Simmons, Lina Fruzetti, Marida Hollos and Kay Warren. Thanks also go to Francoise Hamlin for her mentorship. The students in my fall 2014 Anthropology of China and spring 2015 Bioethics and Culture courses sparked new thinking on several of my arguments. Allison Silverman provided excellent assistance in compiling, formating, and proofreading the final manuscript and preparing it for submission.

It has been a pleasure and honor to work with Stanford University Press. I thank Michelle Lipinski for her guidance and editorial suggestions and her steadfast support of this project, Nora Spiegel for her highly competent editorial assistance and her patience, and two anonymous reviewers whose encouraging and constructive feedback helped the manuscript immeasurably and breathed new life into the project.

Finally, I want to thank my family—past, present, and future—to whom this book is dedicated. I will forever be grateful for the support of my parents, Jane and Bernard Mason, and my sister, Cynthia, and for their willingness to stick by me through many ill-timed trips to China over the past fifteen years. My maternal grandparents, Ethel and Benjamin Spivack, both passed away during my first stint in China in 2001–2003. I hope that the fact that my experience there ended up leading to this book might help in some small way to make up for my absence during their final days. My mother was diagnosed with, was treated for, and recovered from cancer during those early days in China as well. I ask for her forgiveness that I was not present for most of those difficult months either. My paternal grandmother, Florence Mason, passed away a month before I left to do my field research in 2008, and I feel grateful that I was able to be present in her final days as I was unable to do for my other grandparents. My niece, Julianna McLaughlin, was born shortly after I returned from my follow-up research trip in 2010. I thank her for her timing and for being her fun and silly self. I also am extremely grateful for the support and encouragement of my parents-in-law Linda and Patrick McCreless, sister-in-law Erin McCreless, and brothers-in-law William McLaughlin and Brian Wells.

I end by extending my deepest gratitude to my husband, Michael McCreless, and my daughter Clara. I met Mike one week before embarking on my PhD studies in 2005 and married him two months before embarking on my fieldwork in 2008. Mike stood by me every step of the way throughout this process, read countless versions of chapters, and endured a great deal of reclusion and grumpiness. He countered it all with his unending patience, encouragement, and love. His unwavering belief in me and in this project, and his willingness to see it through—even when it meant spending our first year of marriage 10,000 miles apart—made everything possible. Clara tolerated being dragged up and down the East Coast to live in three different cities in her first three years of life, being left for weeks at a time without her mother while I made two solo follow-up trips to China, and being hauled off to many long hours at daycare and grandparents' houses while I furiously finished the manuscript. She did so with the kind of cheerful grace that shouldn't be required of a three-year-old. She is the world to me, and I will forever be grateful.

INFECTIOUS CHANGE

Introduction

After SARS

In February 2003, a Chinese physician crossed the border between Mainland China and Hong Kong and spread a novel influenza-like virus to over a dozen international hotel guests, who then carried it to Toronto, Singapore, and Hanoi. Severe Acute Respiratory Syndrome (SARS) went on to kill about 800 people worldwide and sicken 8,000. Of these, 349 reported deaths and 5,327 cases occurred in China (WHO 2003, 13).

After initially denying the scope of SARS within China, the country's highest leaders admitted error on April 20, 2003, following a whistle-blower's report. Under immense international pressure to contain the outbreak, the central government discharged the Minister of Health and the mayor of Beijing, promised to cooperate with all international disease control efforts, and began encouraging local municipalities to institute aggressive measures to control the outbreak.[1] Measures included quarantining thousands of people, even sealing off entire hospitals, schools, and apartment buildings; rapidly building SARS treatment facilities, including an entire SARS hospital in Beijing in one week; closing down movie theaters, Internet cafes, and other public spaces; setting up neighborhood watch systems to root out potential carriers of the disease; and drowning thousands of civets—suspected animal reservoirs of the SARS virus—in disinfectant. The World Health Organization (WHO) praised China's efforts and credited the Chinese government with playing a critical role in the successful global SARS containment effort (Fidler 2004; Saich 2006).

In Tianmai, a large city located near the epicenter of the initial SARS outbreak in southeastern China's Pearl River Delta region, those who worked in public health faced a period of sudden and intense political and professional pressures unlike any they had ever experienced.* One woman told me, "It was like being a soldier on the frontline of a war." A flu specialist at the Tianmai Center for Disease Control and Prevention (TM CDC) described her experience with SARS this way:

> I worked to the point of crying, worked to the point of *xinku, hen xinku* [bitter hardship]. There was a lot of pressure. As soon as something happened, the leaders would always push you for a result, "What is it? Is it SARS or not?" . . . We were afraid of reporting the wrong thing. . . . So, at the time, our hearts were tired, and our bodies were also tired.

Xiao Lin, a young man who joined the TM CDC just prior to the appearance of SARS, recounted how during the epidemic he worked feverishly all day distributing disinfectant materials.[2] Every few days he also had to take a turn answering a hotline on the night shift. "We couldn't really sleep at all, because we'd maybe doze off and then get a call at one or two in the morning and then have to write up our report," he told me. He said that the TM CDC leaders were so anxious to show that they were putting together a strong response that when he failed to pick up a call one night while he was in the bathroom, the leaders installed a telephone in the bathroom stall to make sure that such an oversight never happened again.

---

*Note that Tianmai is a pseudonym, and certain identifying information about the city has been changed or omitted. Due to certain unique characteristics that were not possible to entirely alter or eliminate, readers familiar with China may have little trouble identifying the true identity of Tianmai. I nevertheless made the decision to use a pseudonym for the city for the purposes of both protecting certain informants from potential political repercussions and keeping a promise to the director of the Tianmai CDC that I would not refer to his center by name in my ethnographic work. However imperfect, the simple act of refraining from naming the city in this book allows all of Tianmai's public health institutions, which all use the city name, to keep their names out of print and also provides some basic, if limited, protections to those who work there.

By July 2003, SARS had disappeared. The profound impact that this brief epidemic had on public health in China, however, had only just begun to take shape. This book tells the story of how the first global health crisis of the twenty-first century transformed a Chinese public health apparatus— once famous for its grassroots, low-technology approach to improving health— into a professionalized, biomedicalized, and globalized technological machine that frequently failed to serve the Chinese people.[3]

The system that under the otherwise deeply problematic leadership of Chairman Mao Zedong nearly doubled life expectancy in the world's largest country had, in the several decades preceding SARS, sunk into unfunded obscurity. Overshadowed by an economic development agenda that left little room for mundane concerns like measles and diarrhea, public health in China became both invisible and ineffective. But in a serendipity of timing, the year that SARS arrived also marked the year that thousands of crumbling Mao-era local public health posts known as Anti-Epidemic Stations (*fangyizhan*) reopened their doors as shiny new Centers for Disease Control and Prevention (CDCs, *jibing yufang kongzhi zhongxin*). The Chinese state had begun in the 1990s to develop the CDCs as part of its vision of establishing a modern, professional research and disease control system—but until SARS hit, local leaders lacked the funds, trained personnel, and political capital to implement this grand vision. SARS provided all of these things, remaking an administrative experiment into a sophisticated new system of disease control and transforming what had been a technical trade into a prestigious biomedical profession.

The new public health profession that emerged had a very different mandate from its Mao-era predecessor. Because the blame initially put on China for the SARS epidemic led to highly public shaming and economic losses for the Chinese Party-state, the motivation to do whatever was necessary to prevent another SARS was extremely strong. And because SARS came onto the scene just as the Chinese state was reinventing its public health system, these motivations, and the mission they implied, became hardwired into the new public health system itself. Local public health in China became geared toward the protection of global, rather than local, interests and toward the protection of a cosmopolitan middle-class dream rather than toward the betterment of the poor.

Chinese public health professionals learned to govern local populations on behalf of what I call the *common*: an idealized world of modernity, science, and trust that they hoped through their work to be able to find abroad and build at home. The separation that arose between the common being served and the populations being governed—what I refer to as the *bifurcation of service and governance*—had significant consequences for the professionalization of public health in China. The potential for this separation to occur anywhere where professionals serve an aggregate also has important implications for the ethics of public health, and global public health, more broadly.

Tianmai, City of Immigrants

Based primarily on thirteen months of ethnographic fieldwork conducted at the TM CDC and other local public health institutions between 2008 and 2010, this book traces the transformation of public health in China after SARS by following the lives of dozens of public health professionals who worked in and around a city that I call Tianmai. Tianmai is located near the border between Mainland China and Hong Kong in China's Pearl River Delta region, in the heart of Guangdong province—the region of China associated with Cantonese culture and language. But Tianmai is not Cantonese. It is, as its residents call it, a "city of immigrants" (*yimin chengshi*). It is a cacophony of cultures, cuisines, and languages from all over China, a medley of high-rise apartment buildings and villages, rice fields and traffic and factories. "We are like a small country," several informants told me. And indeed Tianmai, with approximately 16 million people at the time of my fieldwork, is larger than many small countries.[4] The vast majority of Tianmai's population migrated from the interior of China to search, as the "city of immigrants" mantra suggests, for a better life.

Filling Tianmai's urban villages, luxury hotels, narrow alleyways, and open-air markets are smells from every one of China's cuisines. Hot Sichuan oils sting the nose, steaming Chaozhou seafood arrives at tables straight from tanks that line the first floors of massive restaurants, American-style steaks fill staid dining halls at resort golf courses, and barbecue and beer are served at outdoor picnic tables, as men with long fingernails, moist cigarettes hanging from their mouths, scrape scales from still-flopping fish. There are squares of Hakka tofu with succulent pork in the middle, Hunanese balls of taro in hot sauce, Shanghai dumplings, and Beijing duck. And there are Starbucks and McDonalds and KFCs, Italian bakeries and Irish pubs and pizza with ketchup served as tomato sauce. There are pigeons roasted on sticks and, nestled between high-rises and sprawling for miles at the far ends of the city, there are fields of rice and grazing cattle.

Tianmai was founded in the early 1980s, at the dawn of Deng Xiaoping's economic reforms, on land that at the time was occupied by 30,000 rural villagers. Deng is a hero to middle-class Chinese all over the country, but he is especially revered in Tianmai. A giant billboard carrying his portrait is one of the most recognized landmarks in the city; a stone statue of Deng rises over Tianmai's highest point, standing guard over a spectacular view of the city; and a museum commemorating the city's history devotes several rooms to Deng's accomplishments and his keepsakes. Comparable iconography of Deng's predecessor, Chairman Mao, is noticeably missing: His portrait is absent from the museum, from classrooms, and from public squares, though it still dangles from the occasional taxi dashboard. Tianmai's public health professionals spoke frequently of their bitterness toward Mao. They blamed him for their families' past suffering, for China's overpopulation problem, for what they perceived to be the country's continued relative backwardness, and for the stifling of ideas that still emanated from the direction of Beijing.

Such bitterness toward the Mao years is not unique to Tianmai. Ann Anagnost (1997) has described how educated Chinese everywhere now look at the Mao years "as an irrational derangement of China's 'natural' course of development" (165). But the directness and passion with which Mao was blamed and Deng celebrated in Tianmai were notable. My informants spoke freely and in detail of things I had rarely heard Chinese friends elsewhere speak of so candidly: the madness of the Great Leap Forward and the starvation they or their parents experienced; the godlike cult that surrounded Mao; the hatred that they felt as children when they stared at Mao's portrait in their classrooms back in Hunan and Hebei provinces; and their nightmares of the Cultural Revolution that left them feeling that the fragile stability they had built for themselves and their families might crumble at any moment. When I climbed Plum Mountain with one of my closest Tianmai friends, she demanded that I take a picture in front of Deng's statue to show my respect. "Deng Xiaoping is China's greatest hero," she told me sternly. "If it weren't for him, you wouldn't be allowed to be here."

The border that separates Tianmai and other Pearl River Delta cities from Hong Kong once represented the line between Mao's China and the West.[5] It was a line across which refugees from China swam, climbed, and ran in a slow trickle for thirty years following the Communist victory in 1949 and across which Hong Kong villagers then watched as quiet Mainland rice fields gave way to skyscrapers (Watson 2004). In 1997, British Hong Kong rejoined the People's Republic of China as a "Special Administrative Region," and this line rapidly became one of the most porous borders in the world, with hundreds of thousands of people flowing with relative freedom in both directions every day.

In addition to serving as a destination for millions of Chinese from the interior of China, Tianmai also became an initial Mainland stop for many of the cross-border travelers. It was a place to change currency, buy clothes at Mainland prices, get a foot massage, visit a prostitute, and then go home or onward into the interior. Its mega-malls seemed to flow uninterrupted from the Hong Kong side of the border; its subway system and regional trains ferried Hong Kong travelers rapidly into the Mainland. All that lay between Hong Kong and Tianmai was an increasingly anachronistic wall of customs agents stamping a stream of hundreds of thousands of passports and "cross-border passes" per day.

The stamps in their passports, however, served to remind those who crossed this border that with the "one country, two systems" policy, Hong Kong remained a quasi-foreign land. Instead of suddenly disappearing with reunification, the border between Hong Kong and the Mainland continued to keep people out and keep people in (Berdahl 1999). This ability to exclude and include ensured that the borderlands of Hong Kong and Tianmai would continue to serve as places where national identities were defined (Newendorp 2008).

By the late 2000s, the border between Mainland China and Hong Kong functioned less to control the mobility of people and more to control the mobility of the microbes (and other undesirable things) those people might be carrying. From the time the SARS virus crossed the border into Hong Kong and then spread around the world, Tianmai's public health professionals found themselves on the front lines of China's biosecurity apparatus (Kleinman and Watson 2006). The Hong Kong border took on outsized significance as the site where frightening diseases were likely to pass between China and the rest of the world. Having initially failed to contain SARS, public health professionals throughout the Hong Kong border region were determined to keep future infections from crossing the border into their cities. Thus one of the first sights travelers encountered on either side of the border in the several years following SARS was a foldout table covered with a white cloth and staffed by nurses in loose-fitting masks, who handed out literature with messages like "Prevent Avian Flu!" in English and Chinese. Overhead monitors carried spooling red admonitions warning tourists that they should see a doctor if they felt ill; at times, the nurses pointed menacing fever guns at suspicious foreheads.

From Patriotic Health Campaigns to CDCs

The fever guns at the border were emblematic of a profound shift in how public health efforts were conceptualized and carried out in China after SARS. Understanding this shift requires a foray into recent Chinese history.

The SARS epidemic happened to hit at almost precisely the same time that China's leaders began transitioning their country's public health system from what they referred to as a "Soviet system" of Anti-Epidemic Stations (AESs) to an "American system" of Centers for Disease Control and Prevention (CDCs) (Lee 2004; Yao and Liu 2006). The "Soviet system" (*sulian moshi*), pioneered in the Soviet Union and adopted by Mao in the early 1950s, called for the establishment of basic health posts at each administrative level of government (provincial, municipal, district, and so on) (Sidel and Sidel 1977). The posts were to make use of sanitation inspection and oversight (*jiance, jiandu*) as a means of preventing epidemics (*fangyi*).

The mandate of China's version of the Soviet system was to improve local *gonggong weisheng*, a Chinese term that is now usually translated as "public health" but until recently more accurately described the concept of "public hygiene." Public hygiene encompassed the "Five Hygiene s" (*wu da weisheng*), which promoted sanitation in five locations: schools, "environments" (usually meaning internal air and water quality in hotels and other businesses), food establishments, occupational settings, and places that use or produce radiation (Lu and Li 2006, 2007). Although many of today's public health professionals have degrees from medical schools with specialties in preventive medicine (*yufang yixue*), epidemiology, or biology, *gonggong weisheng* workers for the most part held public hygiene degrees from vocational schools.[6] The goals of public hygiene were explicitly spatial and proximate: Public hygiene was a technical trade that sought to maintain a clean local environment.

In keeping with these goals, one of the primary responsibilities of the early AESs was to provide logistical support for Mao's mass sanitation campaigns, which helped to usher in dramatic improvements to the health of millions of Chinese peasants (Sidel and Sidel 1982; Yao and Liu 2006). During the period of Mao's reign from 1949 to 1976, according to statistics widely cited in the English-language literature, the infant mortality rate in China fell from 200 per 1,000 to 47 per 1,000 live births, life expectancy almost doubled, the common parasitic disease schistosomiasis was brought under control, millions were vaccinated against a wide variety of other diseases, and venereal disease was nearly eliminated (Horn 1969; Chen 1989). These reports of spectacular success have not gone uncontested (Warren 1988), including by my own informants. Yet few would disagree that significant health gains among the poor were in fact made.

In 1952, Mao launched his first Patriotic Health Campaign (*aiguo weisheng yundong*), as part of his pledge to harness the power of the masses to improve the people's health under a slogan of "prevention first" (*yufang weizhi*). Equating the health of the masses with the health of the new nation, Mao's campaigns declared the improvement of public health to be a patriotic duty. According to firsthand accounts of the period, to prevent the spread of disease, Communist officials organized thousands of peasants to pick up vermin one by one with chopsticks, clean schistosomiasis-carrying snail-infested ponds by hand, and even scare sparrows out of trees by banging pots and pans—the last as part of an effort to eliminate the "Four Pests" (mice, flies, mosquitoes, and sparrows) (Horn 1969; Chen 1989).[7] Brothels were closed, and prostitutes were screened and treated for venereal disease before being sent to reeducation camps (Hershatter 1997; Cohen et al. 2000).

The face of this movement was that of the barefoot doctor (*chijiao yisheng*): an ordinary peasant who underwent several weeks or months of training in disease prevention and simple primary care. Barefoot doctors were responsible for maintaining sanitary conditions in the villages; providing basic health education, immunizations, and primary care; and leading Patriotic Health Campaigns. Historians credit them with providing highly accessible, if sometimes substandard, care to an impressively large proportion of China's rural population. The barefoot doctor movement was hailed internationally at the time as a model for WHO's Primary Health Care movement (Navarro 1984).[8] In the 1970s, Mao became the darling of the international health community, as foreign health workers brought back remarkable success stories from their visits to model villages and work units. Long before the U.S. CDC became a model for Chinese public health, Chinese public health became a model for grassroots global health.

Mao's fundamental message was that ordinary people employing basic techniques grounded in the principles of prevention could create greater improvements in their own health than professionals could with their expert knowledge. The campaigns, as Michel Oksenberg (1974) puts it, "express[ed] confidence in the capacity of China's unskilled, uneducated poor to solve their own problems" (152). But this celebration of low-skilled labor had a darker side. During the Cultural Revolution (1966–1976), Mao put into place what Gail Henderson (1993) calls "the most extreme experiment in radical deprofessionalization of the medical profession ever conducted" (185). Trained physicians were persecuted, removed from their positions, and made to perform manual labor. Medical schools were shut down. What the Party instituted in their place was a model for health management that connected Party leaders, via barefoot doctors, directly with "the masses" for the purpose of enacting public health projects. This bypassed the need for either physicians or trained public health professionals, made clinical care an arm of public health, and made public health an arm of political mobilization. Mao claimed his public health successes as victories of the Party-state and a source of strength for his new utopian future.

This source of strength was short lived. Upon Mao's death and the onset of the reform period in the late 1970s, the government's focus turned away from public health and toward an economic growth-driven agenda. AESs were decentralized, defunded, and partially privatized (Hsiao 1995; Dong, Hoven, and Rosenfield 2005; Liu, Yao, and Liu 2006). Over the next thirty years, the proportion of total health expenditures in China provided by the government fell from 32 percent to 16 percent (Wang, Liu, and Chin 2007). The number of people covered by public health insurance schemes plummeted, particularly in the countryside, causing health inequities and medical bankruptcies to soar (cf. Tang et al. 2008). And, according to my informants, the proportion of the budgets of local AESs that were provided by the state fell to less than 40 percent, from nearly 100 percent prior to the reforms. Beginning in 1985, AESs began charging user fees for sanitation and other prevention services (Yu et al. 2001). By 2005, 50 percent of AESs' revenues came from fees for physical exams and other services (Hsiao and Hu 2011). Sanitation inspections of restaurants, hotels, and factories became the AESs' primary work. The local AESs transformed from a publicly funded arm of mass sanitation campaigns into self-funded sanitation police.

Scholars have suggested that these changes contributed to resurgences in schistosomiasis (Sleigh et al. 1998; Cook and Drummer 2004), venereal disease (Cohen et al. 2000; Abrams 2001), hepatitis (Mausezahl et al. 1996), and tuberculosis (Lee 2004), among other infectious diseases. The effects of infectious disease outbreaks were exacerbated by the decentralization of health financing, which weakened vertical lines of communication between local and higher-level health bodies (Liu 2004, 533). Chronic disease incidence also increased rapidly during the reform era. By the mid-2000s, cancers, strokes, diabetes, and cardiovascular conditions affected over 100 million people in China and overtook infectious diseases as China's leading causes of death (Lee 2004; He et al. 2005).

In Tianmai, concerns grew in the late 1990s about the potential for the surge in infectious disease to go global. The Pearl River Delta had for decades been implicated as a source of flu viruses, and the Tianmai AES joined the WHO influenza surveillance program in 1994. When an outbreak of the deadly H5N1 strain of avian influenza occurred in Hong Kong in 1997, killing six people and sickening eighteen, infectious disease specialists began talking about the region as an incubator for the next influenza pandemic (MacPhail 2014). Dr. Peng, a flu specialist at the TM CDC, said of the 1997 outbreak, "That shook up the whole world. WHO sent U.S. CDC people especially to investigate . . . At the time we had never done avian flu; we could barely do human flu. Afterwards we went to Hong Kong for two months and had an exchange. And from that moment on, the central government started to emphasize flu." In 2000, the Ministry of Health (MOH) established a set of flu surveillance networks and came to Tianmai to inspect its capabilities, to make sure it was up to "international standards." Tianmai passed the test. Money began to trickle into Tianmai for flu surveillance and control. But it wasn't until SARS hit that what had been the priority of a small number of flu specialists suddenly became a major global concern. The trickle of flu money became a torrent. The budget for flu surveillance shot up by a factor of ten, and the size of the flu control team doubled.

The immediate effects of SARS were even more dramatic at a national level. When SARS hit, the disintegration of China's public health system suddenly was exposed for all the world to see. Stung by the loss of face that this bad publicity produced, then-President Hu Jintao declared that the improvement of health systems would be a top priority for his government. According to Wang, Liu, and Chin (2007), the central Chinese government invested $1.3 billion in the first four years after SARS in the new CDC system, investing particularly heavily in the creation of a public health emergency surveillance system. Another $1.4 billion was committed to public health more generally. Along with SARS and avian influenza, the control of HIV/AIDS in China became a priority (see Conclusion). The central government accelerated reforms to the clinical health care system after SARS as well, experimenting with health insurance schemes, reinvesting in the hospital system, and attempting to curb abuses and improve the doctor–patient relationship.[9] Even chronic diseases got an infusion of support, though not as much as those who worked with these diseases had hoped. "On the one hand, there has been more money for everything since SARS, including chronic diseases," said a member of the chronic diseases department at a CDC in nearby Guangzhou. "On the other hand, what we do is not an emergency [*yingji*]. If you have diabetes today, you'll still have it tomorrow and next month and next year. It's slow [*man*]—that's why we call it a 'slow disease' [*manxingbing*, "chronic disease" in Chinese]. So because it's slow, it's not as important, and it doesn't get as much attention."

It would be misleading to imply, however, that Hu's post-SARS health reinvestments were a result only of the global embarrassment that accompanied SARS. In the several years prior to 2003, China's central leaders already recognized that they had a problem and began planning an overhaul of the country's disintegrating health infrastructure. A key part of this overhaul was an initiative to professionalize the AESs and transform them into CDCs.[10]

Beginning in 2002, each of the several thousand AESs was split into a "Health Inspection Institute" (*weisheng jiandusuo*) and a "Center for Disease Control and Prevention" (*jibing yufang kongzhi zhongxin*; "CDC") (Lu and Li 2006). The Health Inspection Institutes (HII) took over the bulk of the sanitation inspections that had dominated the work of the AESs since the early 1980s.[11] The CDCs, on the other hand, were to focus on research, on disease prevention and surveillance, and on epidemiological studies of disease prevalence (Lu and Li 2006). The national China CDC opened in July 2002 (Peng et al. 2003; Lee 2004), replacing the Chinese Academy of Preventive Medicine. Local CDCs opened throughout the country in 2002 and 2003.

The former Tianmai City AES officially reopened its doors as the Tianmai City CDC in May 2003, at the height of the SARS epidemic.

The name CDC, an explicit reference to the U.S. CDC in Atlanta, was intended to evoke a highly modern, scientific, and professional ethos—as well as to lend the new system a sense of legitimacy. When Deng Xiaoping called in 1978 for China to expand its capabilities in science and technology as part of the "Four Modernizations," he launched a proscience fervor that equated "science" (*kexue*) with "modernization" (*xiandaihua*) and "economic development" (*jingji fazhan*) (Simon and Goldman 1989; Greenhalgh and Winckler 2005). The CDCs became a belated extension of this proscience fervor.

Shanghai CDC innovators Jing Peng and colleagues (2003) explain, "Different models of public health structures . . . were studied. Among them, the U.S. model is outstanding because the U.S. CDC is widely recognized as one of the world's premier public health institutions. Its strength is its emphasis on prevention, accomplished by the skillful use of two scientific disciplines: epidemiology and laboratory science" (1992). Indeed, Chinese public health professionals from the local to the national level displayed an admiration for the U.S. CDC that bordered on worshipful, and visits to or from the U.S. CDC became instant status symbols. Many of the TM CDC members I knew suggested that the CDC name also lent their work a sense of importance that was more in keeping with what they felt to be China's increasing global dominance: "The term *station* [*zhan*] implied a small place with a few people, and I guess people abroad didn't know what that meant. What does health have to do with a station? There are bus stations, train stations, but there's no epidemic station. This idea about stations is from the Soviet Union. So we changed the name to the American name—*center*. This sounds like something big and important, something that does something," a parasitologist at the TM CDC told me.

The U.S. CDC played no small role in presenting itself as a model for China's new system. By the late 1990s, it had begun to actively train Chinese public health professionals and assist in developing China's disease control capacities (PRC Ministry of Health et al. 2007; U.S. CDC 2009). Many of my informants told me that their greatest hero was Robert Fontaine, a U.S. CDC epidemiologist in Beijing who ran a program called the Field Epidemiology Training Program (FETP). Graduates of FETP went on to take top posts at local CDCs around the country.[12]

SARS, then, did not create the Chinese CDC system. But it did, largely as an accident of timing, coevolve with it—or, as Sheila Jasanoff (2004) puts it, SARS and the CDC system were "co-produced." During the first year or two of the CDCs' development prior to SARS, the call to build a U.S.-style disease control system remained an unfunded and unclear mandate that lacked momentum. Payment-for-service sanitation inspections still made up the bulk of the CDCs' work, and money for the sort of high-tech labs, surveillance systems, and well-trained personnel that the CDC mandate called for was lacking. The new CDCs also lacked a sense of purpose. "No one knew at first how exactly what we were doing was going to be different from the AES, other than that we couldn't issue fines anymore," one informant told me.

SARS provided all of these things: purpose, funding, political support, energy, and a surge in foreign technical support. It also put the nail in the coffin of public hygiene as a model for public health. With its new focus on the urgently mobile, "public health" in China became partially detached from local spaces. As one leader at a district-level CDC in Tianmai told me, "SARS was really scary, and it spread, so we have to stop it, of course . . . But 'public hygiene' mainly deals only with the local . . . So it doesn't affect the world; it affects only one spot right there. But infectious disease spreads everywhere, so it makes sense to emphasize it more."

The reactions of international agencies to SARS were instrumental in globalizing the focus of local public health in China. WHO's revised International Health Regulations (IHR) (WHO 2005a), released two years after SARS, required member states to report within twenty-four hours any "public health emergency of international concern" (PHEIC) detected on their own soil (WHO 2005a). A PHEIC was defined as any "extraordinary public health event which is determined: (i) to constitute a public health risk to other States through the international spread of disease, and (ii) to potentially require an international response" (WHO 2005a).[13] According to these guidelines, deciding whether a disease is an "emergency" is determined primarily by whether it is likely to spread internationally. The Tianmai CDC swiftly adopted this measure of importance in considering which public health problems to prioritize.

A longtime TM CDC member explained the effects of SARS in this way:

At the time, to tell the truth, people thought the CDC's job was giving out vaccines and disinfection, that's all. The whole society knew the CDC [after SARS], knew that we were primarily here for disease control, for acute infectious disease. We have this important position. . . . After SARS, that made clear what the goal of the TM CDC is. What are the goals of the CDC? What kind of work do we do? This is where the fundamental change came in . . . Now primarily what we do is . . . gradually building preparations, contingency for sudden public health incidents, as well as some infectious disease response.

China's public health professionals finally knew *what* they were supposed to be doing, and they had the resources to do it. But *why* were they doing it? And *who* would benefit?

Defining a Profession, Serving a "Group"

January 5, 2009, The Fifth Annual Spring Festival Performance of the Tianmai CDC system[14]

The lights go up on ten men in white vests with the green TM CDC logo across the back, running onto the stage, arms pumping in unison at their sides, heads bent purposefully. Projected on the screen behind them are buildings crumbling, dirty children crying, desperate mothers reaching out. And then, as if in response to the mothers' pleas, four-foot-tall white characters rise across the screen: "yong women de aixin gei nimen liliang" (draw on our compassion to give you strength). The men disappear, and a beautiful woman dressed in a red and white silk dress hobbles onto the stage with a crutch, her leg buried inside her dress giving the illusion that it has been removed, apparently lost in the Sichuan earthquake. Her bleached-white face is full of dramatic expressions of pain. One of the men rushes back on stage as the music swells, and the montage of destruction on the screen behind him gives way to rescue, muddy men with disinfectant machines strapped to their backs, spraying the threat of disease out of demolished buildings—a symbol of hope.

The woman collapses into the caring TM CDC worker's arms with an expression of abandon and relief. Then she and her rescuer begin to dance, the man swirling her on one foot with surprising grace, and soon there are a half dozen other women on stage in flowing red and white dresses, swaying from side to side, flanked by their CDC rescuers. The women kneel on the ground and begin rising like flowers, as green shoots rise on the screen behind them, disaster giving way to rebirth, Sichuan rising again with the help of the heroes of the TM CDC. Across the screen eight more characters flash: "zhongzhi chengcheng, shouhu Wenchuan" (in union there is strength, guard over Wenchuan [Sichuan]).

An hour later, a 120-person choir drives home the point in song:

you yizhong ai bu xuyao yuyan	There is a kind of love that doesn't need words
wo de kuaile, ni de jiankang	My happiness is your health
you yizhong qing bu qidai lijie	There's a type of kindness that doesn't expect understanding
wo de xingfu, ni de ping'an	My good fortune is your safety
renshenglu manman	The road of life is long and boundless
xieshou fengyu yangfan	Sailing through a rainstorm hand in hand
yong suoyou de fuchu	Sparing no expense
bawo shengming hangchuan	Grasping firmly onto the lifeboat
renshenglu manman	The road of life is long and boundless
wo hui xiangban yongyuan	I will accompany you forever
yong wuyan de shouhu	Silently guarding
jingcai meili renjian	The beautiful and brilliant world of people
yong wuyan de shouhu	Silently guarding
jingcai meili renjian	The beautiful and brilliant world of people

On May 12, 2008, a new emergency provided an occasion for the fledgling CDC system to flex its muscles. A 7.9 magnitude earthquake hit Sichuan province in southwestern China, killing at least 69,000 people in the county of Wenchuan and the surrounding region, leaving millions homeless, and threatening to spread infectious disease. Public health professionals from around the country, along with scores of other government workers, emergency responders, and ordinary citizens, rushed to the scene. "Within twenty-four hours everyone [in the media] was there, showing how bad it was. And our CDC went there, mostly for the after-period [*houqi*] because of the risk of infectious diseases . . . Everyone knew what they were supposed to do," said one woman who had just arrived at the TM CDC when the earthquake hit. "Because it was all clear after SARS."

Yunxiang Yan (2009) describes how a new spirit of volunteerism seemed to sweep over ordinary Chinese when the earthquake struck in Sichuan. Televised human interest stories described heroic acts by first responders and others who selflessly risked all to save strangers: a policewoman who saved hungry orphans by serving as an impromptu wet nurse, a schoolteacher who managed to evacuate all fifty of his students just before his school collapsed.

The local Tianmai public health professionals who rushed off to Sichuan after the earthquake were not acting out of spontaneous volunteerism, however. Ever since the SARS epidemic, they had been actively preparing to respond to China's next big emergency. Unlike the celebrated volunteers who assisted in dramatic rescues, in facing these emergencies public health professionals had few opportunities to pull children from rubble. Armed with backpacks full of disinfectant spray, they were searching for epidemics to prevent, not people to save.

This distinction—between preventing and saving, between stopping the spread of disease and stopping illness in individuals—would become critical to how the profession of public health defined its scope, its mission, and its ethics in China after SARS. According to Chinese public health scholar Hu Runhua, the responsibilities of a public health professional are clear— and are limited. "Public health is to protect and prevent disease in the group (*qunti*)," he wrote in 2003.[15] "If there is an infectious disease outbreak, the hospitals provide treatment; public health should find the source, confirm the reasons for spread, control the transmission channels. *Treatment targets the individual, prevention targets the group*" (134; emphasis added). Definitions like Hu's established a division of labor that created narrow boundaries around the responsibilities of public health professionals in China. As TM CDC members sang in their Spring Festival song, they "silently guard[ed] the beautiful and brilliant world of people"—but contrary to the dramatic reenactments in their performances, they did not save individual persons. Instead, once a problem materialized in the form of a tangible sick person, they wiped themselves clean of professional responsibility.

My interlocutors at the TM CDC defended this strict division of labor— formalized in the Chinese medical education system as the difference between "clinical" (*linchuang*) and "preventive" (*yufang*) medicine—as being entirely in keeping with "international standards."[16] In many ways they were right. The professionalization process in Tianmai after SARS mirrored similar processes that played out over a century ago in other countries. Historical studies of the development of public health in the United Kingdom (Acheson and Fee 1991; Lewis 1991; Porter 1991), the United States (Rosenkrantz 1972, 1974; Rosen 1993; Brandt and Gardner 2000), and France (Barnes 1995, 2006) have shown the ways in which public health and medicine split into distinct disciplines and distinct professions. They also have shown the ways in which public health transitioned in these countries from a broad interdisciplinary effort to improve social welfare and sanitation to a branch of the health sciences with its own accreditation, ethical codes, professional norms, and methodologies.[17] What distinguished public health from medicine in these accounts was the focus on prevention as opposed to cure and on populations as opposed to individuals (Brandt and Gardner 2000). Public health professionals were responsible for the group, leaving it to their physician colleagues to worry about the individual clinical encounter.

Promising service to the "group" only, however, turned out to be as evasive as it was significant. Lawrence Gostin (2002) notes that, unlike in the case of medicine or law, the aggregate nature of the "client" of public health professionals makes it difficult to pin down exactly what public health professionals' responsibilities are:

> To whom do public health professionals owe a duty of loyalty, and how can these professionals know what actions are morally acceptable? Physicians, attorneys, and accountants have a fiduciary duty to their clients that informs their moral world . . . In the context of public health, the community might be regarded as the "client." The problem is that it is unclear what constitutes a "community"; the notion is often vague and fragmented. (11)

Gostin raises the question of whether it is possible for public health professionals to develop the same kind of clear ethical responsibility to a community that physicians have to their patients or lawyers to their clients. I will suggest in this book that, although it is possible to do so, it is also difficult because of at least three ways in which serving an aggregate—whether a "community" or a "beautiful and brilliant world of people"—is fundamentally different from serving a person.

First, ethical engagement with an aggregate—especially the kind of abstract, statistically based aggregate with which many public health professionals around the world today engage—is not grounded in the kind of one-on-one human contact and "human feelings" (*renqing*) that lie at the core of any empathic response and also serve as fundamental building blocks of Chinese sociality (see Chapter Two). In the course of their work, Tianmai's public health professionals actively distanced themselves from interacting with their clients as subjects, through the building of numerous boundaries between themselves and their target populations and through the avoidance of situations in which they would have to engage with the subjectivity of the people who made up those populations (see Chapters One and Three).

Second, the slippery edges of "community" open the door for public health professionals to be able to leave out from this category those whom they feel they cannot or should not let in. As I will discuss in Chapter One, my informants' commitments to serving the "group" allowed for a slippage that left out from that group most of the individuals who actually lived in Tianmai.

Finally, in China, as in many places, most of the institutions where public health professionals work are, directly or indirectly, arms of the state. The TM CDC is a government-affiliated *"shiye danwei,"* or "technical work unit" (Lu and Perry 1997, 6–7).[18] Only the local Bureau of Health (BOH, now the Health and Family Planning Commission) has the power to hire and fire TM CDC personnel, and by 2010 the TM CDC's budget was almost entirely dependent once again on BOH funding.[19] Local government directives largely determined the daily work in which the TM CDC engaged. In short, though technically independent, public health professionals at the TM CDC were essentially government employees, and they were seen as such by the general public, which usually grouped the TM CDC with the rest of the local government (*zhengfu*) (Tomba 2014).

Clinicians who work for public hospitals in China also work for the state. But, as Gostin (2002) points out, because clinicians are charged with healing tangible individuals, a clear dyadic relationship establishes unity between the client being targeted and the client being served. In the context of a doctor-patient relationship, although physicians sometimes violate the ethical norms of the clinical relationship, those norms establish clear expectations: A physician may *work* for the state, but his or her primary professional *responsibility* should be to the patient being treated. A doctor who treats a patient's illness is *supposed* to be doing so for the benefit of that same patient (even if this sometimes does not happen; see Blumenthal and Hsiao 2015). The state might manage how this happens and how much the clinician is paid, but the intended recipient of the service is clear.

In abstracting the "patient" to the group, however, the relationship is no longer dyadic and the identity of the service recipient no longer clear. A local public health professional has a responsibility to guard the interests of the state by *governing* local populations that may spread diseases. Thus he or she is always in some sense serving the state. But his or her object of *professional* service—the client group that the public health professional considers to be his or her "patient"—can vary, and the recipients of any benefits produced through the governance of infectious populations may not be the same as the participants in the governance exercise itself. That is, the "patient" who is treated may not be the same as the "patient" who receives the benefit of that treatment. The group being served is not always equivalent to the group being governed.

During an epidemic outbreak, for example, on behalf of the state a public health professional might very reasonably quarantine one group of people (for example, those who flew on a plane with a confirmed case of novel influenza) for the benefit of another (those who live in the city where the plane has landed). In one sense the quarantine represents public health's privileging of the group over the individual, as the people on the flight are obligated to forego their individual freedoms temporarily so that the city might remain disease free and avoid the social instability or economic harm that can come with an infectious outbreak. But even at the level of the group we can see that there is an imbalance of cost and benefit: One group (those on the plane) is sacrificing for another (those in the receiving city). The group being quarantined will not necessarily benefit from the quarantine, even at a group level; in some cases, most or even all members of the group might be harmed (for example, through increased likelihood of exposure to those already infected, suspension of freedoms, mental health ramifications, threat to employment, and so on). Still, in this case, protecting the unexposed group is deemed more important. The group being targeted and the group being protected are necessarily *not* one and the same.

What may make this seem fair and reasonable is that the distinction between the group that is served and the group that has to sacrifice is in theory circumstantial and temporary. That is, public health professionals ostensibly made the distinction based on the epidemiological pattern of the particular outbreak and not on any inherent characteristics of the groups themselves. Those individuals making up the group being sacrificed in the name of a larger common good, the theory goes, may well benefit the next time, when others might need to sacrifice their freedoms to protect *them*. There is no systematic rule that governs the distinction between subgroups that may emerge under specific circumstances (Bayer and Fairchild 2004).

But this only works if the chances of being in the sacrificial group versus the benefiting group are equal for all—a proposition that rarely plays out in real life. In their description of cholera control measures during an outbreak in Venezuela, for example, Briggs and Mantini-Briggs (2003) describe how indigenous people marked as "unsanitary subjects" were quarantined to protect the region's "sanitary citizens." It was unthinkable in the classist and racist context in which they worked that the reverse would ever occur. Adia Benton (2014) describes echoes of this same principle in the state-imposed quarantines of Liberian slums and Sierra Leonian villages during the 2014 Ebola outbreak (see also McNeil 2014; Onishi 2014). As I will show in Chapter Four, the 2009 H1N1 influenza outbreak exhibited more subtle but similar biases: Certain groups were seen as inherently more obligated to sacrifice than others. Underlying all of these cases is the unspoken assumption that some people (wealthy, white, "civilized") are more worth saving than others (poor, nonwhite, "backward"). The latter groups are perpetually seen as sources of disease, whereas the former are its victims.

The SARS incident reflected these types of divisions. The disease arose in China and spread to the rest of the world; the patient-group to be "treated" through strict, decisive governance (Chinese, especially those who engaged in backward eating practices; see Chapter Four) became distinct from the patient-group to be served (the rest of the world, especially the "civilized" Western world). The Chinese Party-state tacitly endorsed this view: Becoming a good global health citizen through the aggressive control of potentially diseased populations at home became a means for the state to gain greater global power (Fidler 2004; Saich 2006). Thus, for Tianmai's public health professionals, fulfilling their duties to the state meant *governing* dangerous local populations to *serve* "the rest of the world." This separation that arose between the group being served and the group being governed resulted in what I call the *bifurcation of service and governance*.

As I noted earlier, however, the boundaries of groups are inherently fluid. The new, highly educated public health professionals who came to the TM CDC after SARS—many of whom were educated abroad in Western contexts—aspired to be members of the patient-group to be served. They were not part of the "backward" Chinese who needed to be governed to prevent SARS, they told me; rather, they *should* be part of the (modern, cosmopolitan, civilized) client-group that stood to benefit. And the potential benefits of being a client, as my interlocutors saw it, went far beyond the bounds of protected biological health, to include economic, lifestyle, and moral gains. By effectively serving their client-group, Tianmai's public health professionals hoped to one day receive the myriad benefits of their own service.

Defining the "Common" in China

My interlocutors in Tianmai told me that the group focus of public health came naturally to them because of the collectivist nature of "Chinese culture." Westerners, they told me, worry about individual rights, whereas Chinese worry about what is best for the group. But the assumption that Chinese society is or always has been a collectivist one oriented around achieving a common good represents a partial truth at best (Yan 2003; Steele and Lynch 2012). It is true that individualism per se is fairly new in China—but collectivism is fairly new, too, and has radically morphed in recent years. The particular nature of the group obligations that Chinese public health professionals accepted in the 2000s emerged from this complex history.

In the 1930s, Fei Xiaotong, the founding father of Chinese sociology, developed a set of influential theories about the fundamental relationships that pattern Chinese sociality (1980, 1992). Fei described how traditional Chinese society was built out of interconnected webs of dyadic relationships (*guanxi wang*) steeped in "human feelings" (*renqing*) that established sets of reciprocal obligations between partners in the relationship (see also Yang 1994; Yan 1996; Kipnis 1997). These *guanxi* relationships provided a basis for ethical engagement (based in Confucian principles of *ren* and *li*; see Chapter Two) and served as a primary source of material and emotional support. Fei (1992) noted that a community could expand and contract based on the particularities of the relationships of the people involved; he compared this to "circles that appear on the surface of a lake when a rock is thrown into it," with each rock corresponding to an ego (62–63). In Fei's China there was no "common good"—each ego's universe was unique and impermanent.

One of Chairman Mao's most ambitious goals was to remove kin and *guanxi* obligations and replace them with a principle of absolute loyalty to the Party. Mao communized villages, outlawed lineage loyalties and ancestor worship, and attempted to break down the basic family unit. Interpersonal relationships between subjects were no longer supposed to constitute the nexus of Chinese sociality; under Maoism, relationships with individual others did not matter any more. Only loyalty to the Party and a commitment to "serve the people" (*wei renmin fuwu*) were important. Haiyan Lee (2014) describes how the Party disrupted what Zygmunt Bauman calls the "moral party of two": As individuals became subsumed by the "people" (*renmin*), the ethical response to the intersubjective encounter between two *guanxi* partners was replaced by the religion-like ethics of the Party (21). Lee writes, "The People-as-One admitted no internal division. There was no 'in-between' and hence no possibility of genuine friendship; there was only the aesthetic intimacy of camaraderie eulogized as sublime socialist solidarity" (23). The "people" were like the children of God, the recipients of the good of a benevolent paternalistic state (Cho 2013). They were both the Party-state's servants and the objects of service: To "serve the people" was to "serve the Party." And to serve the Party was to serve the common good.

Mobilizing the people to serve the common good was often described as mobilizing the "masses" (*qunzhong*)—a term that evoked an image of a face-less, undifferentiated crowd. "Mobilizing the masses" meant mobilizing the Chinese people to act as a single, unified force. Mao's public health work, especially his Patriotic Health Campaigns, depended on the brute force of millions of people working tirelessly together and thus leaned heavily on this imagery of the masses.

After the Chinese government launched its dramatic national campaign in 2003 to control the SARS epidemic, international observers praised this effort as a positive vestige of Maoist mass mobilizations (Kaufman 2006, 2008). Chinese public health experts and historians also embraced this view (Li and Deng 2004), arguing that government-led, Mao-style mass campaigns were important tools for stemming emerging infectious diseases and preventing associated economic destruction (Zhang et al. 1998; Ai 2003; Chen, Xu, and Tan 2004; Xiao 2005; Luo et al. 2006). Some of the post-SARS rhetoric from the central government urged a renewed role for mass mobilizations, as well as a renewed focus on "the people's health" (*renmin jiankang*). In a widely cited address to the National Health Work Conference on July 28, 2003, Vice Premier Wu Yi, who led China's aggressive SARS response, declared: "Building public health requires government, society, organizations, and the masses' widespread participation and mutual effort. The government especially needs to . . . organize all walks of life and the large-scale masses to work together to face emergency outbreak situations and infectious disease epidemics."[20]

My informants insisted, however, that Wu Yi's suggestion that mass mobilizations could continue to drive public health work in China was based on a set of false assumptions: that the "masses" were still mobilizable, that the state was still a benevolent provider for the "people," and that a Party-led vision of the state could still represent the "common good." But by the time SARS arrived in 2003, neither the "masses" nor the "people"—at least as Mao conceived them—were anywhere to be found, and few believed in Mao's original vision for the common good. Beginning after the death of Mao, the "people" had become bound up once again in webs of interpersonal relationships. The family and village had returned as important anchors of community life, and the interpersonal relationship based in *guanxi* and *renqing* had returned as a central organizing principle. As cities became more diverse and crowded, city dwellers relied on *guanxi*, steeped in commonalities like hometown, school ties, or language, to provide them with security, access to goods, and a sense of belonging.

To the extent that they still existed as a coherent group, the "people" of twenty-first-century China were more mobile than those of Mao's time, less bound together by a common set of values and ideologies, and more likely to profess Deng Xiaoping's mantra of "to get rich is glorious" than Mao's mantra of "serve the people." Though they remained patriotic, their patriotism was not usually directed toward the Party (see Hoffman 2010). They also were more economically diverse and internally divided. A thriving middle class and a growing class of superrich seemed disinterested in service of any kind. In the new era, a worker at a community health service center told me, "You do not serve the people [*wei renmin fuwu*], you serve the money [*wei renminbi fuwu*]."[21] Mun Young Cho (2013) describes in her ethnography of laid-off workers in Northeastern China how, when the state retreated from its paternalistic role in providing for the everyday lives of workers and peasants, the Party stopped serving the people. It should not be surprising, then, that the people also stopped serving the Party.

Out of the ashes of Mao's Communist fervor and the people's waning reverence for the Party grew new possibilities for a "common good" to be served. In the realm of public health, the "common" indexed by the concept of the "common good" took on a number of forms.[22] No longer bound by Patriotic Health Campaigns, given the education and opportunity to take on leadership roles as "experts" once more, public health professionals after SARS held on to certain elements of Mao-era utopianism, but they set their sights well beyond the Party-state. Their new common as they conceived it was, broadly, the "beautiful and brilliant world of people"—a concept that conjured not "the people" in Mao's sense but rather an idealized dream of a modern, "civilized" society rooted in science, rationality, stability, and trust that they hoped through their work to be able to find abroad and build at home. Included in this common were Western partners as well as certain types of Chinese (the middle-class citizen, the transnational scientist, the well-educated professional). Rural migrants, the "backward," and the insufficiently educated were excluded. The Party-state and its interests lurked behind the common, but for my interlocutors the state was more often seen as an obstacle and a nuisance rather than an object of service itself. Tianmai's public health professionals worked for the state, but their goal was to *serve* the common.

Each chapter of this book follows my interlocutors as they attempted to serve one or more instantiations of the common. Chapter One looks at Tianmai's public health professionals' efforts to serve a *civilized immigrant common* of virtuous immigrants; Chapter Two considers how they attempted to build a *professional common* of local public health professionals; Chapter Three focuses on how public health professionals tried to serve, and eventually join, a *transnational scientific common* of scientific researchers; and Chapter Four takes on their efforts to serve both a *global health common* of global health practitioners and a *global common* of modern, civilized people around the world.

What united the various iterations of the common was their dreamlike nature. The common was always an ideal type (Schutz 1967; Weber 1978)—an imaginary of the professional, the scientist, the cosmopolitan Chinese—that rarely matched up with reality. This space between imaginaries and realities became a constant source of disappointment for Tianmai's public health professionals as they discovered that the groups that they so desperately wanted to call their own were not quite what they imagined them to be.

Serving, Governing, and (Mis)Trusting

The primary tool that Tianmai's public health professionals had at their disposal for serving the common was the effective *governance* of local populations. But governing the population was a trickier proposition than it seemed. By the time SARS arrived, exercising the sort of biopolitical control characteristic of Mao-era governance had become extremely difficult, and the question of who or what—if not the "masses" or the "people"—public health professionals should or even *could* be governing was not a trivial one.

During the Mao period, to facilitate mobilization and control, peasant masses were organized into communes, whereas in cities the worker masses were organized into work units (*danwei*), which formed bounded urban communities that were (and still are) often physically gated off (cf. Bray 2006). But the communes steadily broke up throughout the 1980s, and *danweis*—though still important forms of community for many, including members of the TM CDC—no longer functioned as the single bounded work and living spaces they once were. The Party's control over *danweis* also began to weaken: At the TM CDC, for example, the power of the Party Secretary become largely ceremonial, as he ceded control to the more highly trained CDC director (*zhuren*). Many middle-class residents moved out of *danwei* housing into private gated residencies (*xiaoqu*), where they actively seized control over their own living spaces through self-governance (Zhang 2010; Tomba 2014).

Dr. Shu, a longtime member of the TM CDC vaccination department, summed up the reform-era public health governance problem this way:

> Yes, [Mao vaccinated a lot of people] but that's only because at the time you got to a village and they would just round everyone up and do it—it was very efficient. Not like now when people don't listen, and the population is too mobile, you can't just make a proclamation and organize a large-scale thing anymore.... Now people don't listen [*ting hua*], they think "*wo meiyou shenme bing, da zhen gan ma?*" [I'm not sick, what are you doing vaccinating me?].

What public health professionals were left with in the 2000s was a mishmash of relatively ineffective administrative means with which to manage the diseases of a mobile, diverse, and uncooperative populace. In Tianmai, this was a daunting task indeed. TM CDC members were responsible for governing the health of all of Tianmai's then-16 million residents—a task that seemed impossible. What felt somewhat more plausible was determining which groups of residents posed the greatest threat of launching something like SARS and then focusing on attempting to govern those. These threatening aggregates of potential infection made up what my informants commonly referred to as the "population" (*renkou*).

In one sense, the "population" simply represents any target object of public health. Epidemiologists and other trained public health professionals in the West frequently conceive of their work as dealing in "populations"—that is, large groups of people the parameters and characteristics of which are statistically determined by the particular project in question. Having embraced the scientific view of public health, Chinese public health professionals readily embraced the idea of dealing in "populations" (*renkou*).

Renkou took on special resonance in China, however, in part because in the 1980s it became the object of governance for the so-called one-child policy, the decades-long birth control campaign that limited most families to one or two children.[23] Greenhalgh and Winckler (2005) define *population* (*renkou*), as it was used in this campaign, as a "biological entity dictating an approach to governance guided by science" (285). Cho (2013) shows how the construction of this *renkou* entity, which also turned up in all sorts of places outside the realm of birth control, stripped the urban poor of their exalted Mao-era status as "the people" and transformed them into a group to be enumerated and managed just like any other population in the world. As a "population," "the people" became "numbers without history," Cho (2013) argues—a "collective form of grouping that renders focused research, measurement, and intervention possible" (70).

Greenhalgh and Winckler (2005) show how, after focusing on the numbers and measurement side of *renkou* during the early years of the one-child policy, the government transitioned in the 1990s and 2000s to attempting to maximize population "quality" via the self-regulation of Chinese subjects (see also Foucault 1990). But when talking about *renkou* in the context of their public health work, Tianmai's public health professionals usually were referring to groups of low-quality (*suzhi di*) people whom they felt were incapable of self-regulation or of quality improvement. The population was biologically and numerically dangerous; the term almost always implied a problem to be solved, rather than a resource to be maximized.

The biggest population problem (*renkou wenti*) that my interlocutors felt they had to solve was the problem of the floating population (*liudong renkou*) of rural-to-urban migrants, who in their large quantities and low quality threatened to spread disease and spark chaos. Though the floating population was not the only population of concern, it was by far the largest. Public health professionals expended a lot of effort trying to control it—but relatively little effort trying to serve it.

This does not mean they wanted to cause the floating population harm. The great majority of my informants had no ill will for rural migrants. And the great majority of them were kind people committed to building a better China. As striving middle-class Chinese, Tianmai's public health professionals were very much a part of the neoliberal waves of "individuation" (Ong and Zhang 2008) and "individualization" (Yan 2009) that swept through China in the 1990s and 2000s, whereby personal self-development overtook loyalty to family or country as motivating factors behind major life pursuits (though country remained important; see Hoffman 2010). But, at the same time, they were working in an occupation with a long history of service, and Tianmai's public health professionals took the call to service seriously. These were not purely selfish neoliberal subjects devoid of any purpose beyond their own gain. Instead they had, as Kleinman and colleagues (2011) put it, a "pro-social moral core" (11). They were on a mission to serve someone. That someone was just usually not the same someone that they were attempting to govern.

The bifurcation of service and governance that resulted fed patterns of *social mistrust* in China (Yan 2009). Social and political theorists have long pegged China as a "low-trust society" (Fukuyama 1995) because of its kin- and *guanxi*-based sociality dependent on personalistic trust between intimates (see Chapter Two). Yunxiang Yan (2009) defines "social trust"—what he sees as the antidote to the low-trust society—as "a more generalized trust in social institutions that will behave in accordance with the stated rules; in experts who will guard the rules to make the institutions work well; and also in strangers who will work for peaceful and non-harmful social interactions" (285). Social trust was about trusting that money paid would produce an agreed-upon service, that food purchased would have only the ingredients listed on the package, and that cars would stop at red traffic lights.

My informants frequently told me that they trusted in none of these things. And they did not think that anyone (collaborators, superiors, subordinates, or the general public), other than their own kin and *guanxi* partners, trusted *them*. This made it exceedingly difficult to work with colleagues to build the *professionalized trust* that they told me was necessary to make their profession more scientific (see Chapter Two). The public, meanwhile, (often with good reason) did not trust that public health professionals were acting in service of Tianmai people (see Chapters One and Three). Feeling that they were lacking in the ability to build trust with strangers either inside or outside their workplaces, my interlocutors fell back on familiar patterns of personalistic trust embedded in *guanxi* relationships. And yet this only exacerbated problems of mistrust. Drawing on *guanxi* to accomplish public health tasks reinforced the feeling among the public and even among each other that those completing the tasks were more concerned with fulfilling the expectations of *guanxi* relationships than with providing a service.

One of the most consistent attributes that Tianmai's public health professionals imagined the *common* to have was this missing element of trust. My interlocutors expressed great certainty that if they could only fight their way into membership in the transnational scientific common, if they could only be truly accepted into a global common, if they could only build a true professional common in their own public health system, then they would finally be able to trust and be trusted. But this promised land of trust always shimmered like a mirage, just beyond their grasp. No matter how well they tried to serve the common, trust continued to elude them.

Doing Fieldwork in Tianmai

Prior to the start of my fieldwork, foreign and Chinese scholars alike warned me not to conduct research in Tianmai. They told me that anything I learned there would be too esoteric to be of relevance to the rest of China. Tianmai, they told me, is not "real" China. It is too new, too wealthy, too close to Hong Kong, and too far from Beijing. It cannot tell you anything about how things really are in China—China for them usually meaning Beijing, Shanghai, or the rural heartland.

But what could be a better place to see the Chinese heartland than a place where thousands of different pieces of that heartland have converged? What would be a better place to understand the breathless pace of change that the reform era has brought to China than a city that exploded from village to metropolis in thirty years? As a display at Tianmai's municipal history museum proudly asserts (in English), "Tianmai exhibits to the world the vigor and bright future of socialist China." Although there is no one place in China that can represent the country as a whole, if there were such a place surely it would be this hodgepodge of Chinas all rolled into one.

Still, it is true that Tianmai represents an unusual case study for understanding local public health, in China or elsewhere. As a brand new city, it is a seemingly blank canvas on which public health professionals (and others) are able to project their preferred images of themselves. As a new immigrant city, it has no entrenched local residents against whom invading migrants can be pitted, as is so common in nativist discourses elsewhere; the rationales for the exclusion of migrants must be constructed in other ways (Markel 1997; Shah 2001; Willen 2007). Finally, situated as it is on the border between Hong Kong (China's "Gateway to the World") and the Pearl River Delta (supposed incubator of new influenza strains), Tianmai provides an environment in which a global common can easily be envisioned, local threats quickly become recognizable as global threats, and the specter of infectious ruin looms large.

All of these factors make Tianmai an excellent place to study the twenty-first-century public health imaginary because they accentuate, exaggerate, and render visible dynamics that are present all over China and all over the world—but too often remain buried. Following James Ferguson (1994), I argue that seemingly odd cases can sometimes be the best ones for drawing out widely applicable points. Discrimination against migrants and the poor is ubiquitous in every corner of the world; connections to the global in a postmodern world are everywhere inescapable. Tianmai simply lays these dynamics bare.

I came to Tianmai by accident. I originally planned to base my research in Guangzhou—also located in the Pearl River Delta—where I lived for two years in the early 2000s as an English teacher. But after a summer of failed attempts to gain permission to conduct long-term research in Guangzhou, I fled to Hong Kong, where I received my first piece of positive advice about Tianmai: Try going there. It is open and modern, and they would be willing to talk to you, I was told. What's more, Tianmai was ahead of the curve in implementing a broad range of programs and reforms, so I would get to see the future of public health in China by working there. And so in the summer of 2007 I attended a banquet in a hotel at a beach resort on the eastern edge of Tianmai, and, after drinking plenty of *baijiu* and building some *guanxi* of my own, I was invited to visit the Tianmai CDC and meet with the influenza surveillance team. A week later the director of the CDC invited me to do my fieldwork at his institution.

I rotated to ten of the TM CDC's nineteen nonadministrative departments between September 2008 and August 2009, participating in the daily activities and research projects of each one and interviewing department members.[24] My participant observation activities included working with department members in their offices; going with them to lower-level CDCs as they negotiated support for public health projects; assisting with project implementation, outbreak investigations, and sanitation inspections; volunteering in the outpatient clinic; and translating promotional materials and scholarly articles into English. In addition, I interviewed the department heads of almost all twenty-four departments at the TM CDC, as well as the center leaders, and I participated in centerwide events. I conducted a month of follow-up fieldwork at the TM CDC in August 2010 and another four weeks of follow-up research in January and August 2014.

To supplement my work at the TM CDC, I conducted several interviews and one day of participant observation at four of the six district-level CDCs in Tianmai and longer periods of participant observation and interviewing at the other two. I also conducted interviews at ten "street-level" (*jiedao*) CDCs, five community health service centers (*shequ jiankang fuwu zhongxin*), several hospitals, two maternal and child health centers, two vaccination stations, and several administrative offices of the Tianmai BOH. In addition, I conducted interviews with leaders and department heads at the following city-level public health institutions: the Tianmai Center for Chronic Disease Prevention and Control (CCDC), the Tianmai Food and Drug Administration (TM FDA), the Tianmai Health Inspection Institute, the Tianmai Health Education Research Center, the Tianmai Mental Health Center, and the Tianmai Occupational Health Institute.

I conducted supplementary ethnographic research in the neighboring city of Guangzhou, where I spent approximately one-quarter of my fieldwork time.[25] My work in Guangzhou provided both context and contrast to my work in Tianmai. Guangzhou is similar in size to Tianmai, is also wealthy and full of migrant workers, and also played a pivotal role in the SARS epidemic of 2003. The reforms occurring there were similar to those I observed in Tianmai. Unlike Tianmai, however, Guangzhou is an ancient city with a dominant local Cantonese population. The average age in Guangzhou is much higher than in Tianmai, and though after SARS the focus on infectious disease, pandemic preparedness, and research was similar to that in Tianmai, attention to chronic disease was greater in Guangzhou.

In Guangzhou I conducted multiple interviews and brief periods of participant observation with the Guangzhou CDC (GZ CDC), several Guangzhou district-level CDCs, the Guangdong Provincial CDC, several Guangzhou hospitals, and the public health school of a major university in Guangzhou, where I attended classes and accompanied students as they completed their research projects (see Chapter Three). The university was a feeder school for both the Guangzhou and Tianmai CDCs and so became a good choice for studying the educational backgrounds and trajectories of Tianmai's public health professionals.

I also made site visits and conducted interviews in Beijing at the national-level China CDC and several of its associated institutes, as well as at two universities in Beijing and at a number of foreign organizations with head-quarters in Beijing, including the U.S. CDC, WHO, the United Nations Programme on HIV and AIDS (UNAIDS), and two major NGOs. In Hong Kong I conducted interviews at three universities and at the Hong Kong Centre for Health Protection, which was established in the wake of SARS.

My access to the TM CDC was made possible through the support of the center's director, whom I call Director Lan. As one interlocutor put it, "If Director Lan hadn't said so, no one would talk to you." At the TM CDC I shared an office with Lan's wife, who also set up most of my formal inter-views, arranged my rotation schedule, and even cared for me when I fell sick; she became a very good friend. I ate lunch in the cafeteria and made friends with other employees. My access at the other Tianmai locations was facili-tated through the *guanxi* of my colleagues at the TM CDC. My access to the Guangzhou locations was facilitated through a key contact at the university in Guangzhou. A broad network of connections built up through years of living and working in southeastern China connected me with contacts in Beijing and Hong Kong.

The TM CDC was an ideal place to study the development of the pub-lic health profession in China after SARS. Although it had especially high levels of funding, training, and infrastructure development compared with other local CDCs, it also stood at the leading edge of national public health reforms and presented a model that other cities were trying to emulate. And while the CDC was only one of dozens of public health institutions in Tian-mai, it was the most prestigious and, according to public health professionals I interviewed at other institutions, the most "professional" (*zhuanye*) of the major public health institutions in Tianmai.

The city level is a particularly relevant unit of study for understanding the decentralized process through which systemic reforms progress in China. Under China's system of "fragmented authoritarianism," local governments take on a high degree of autonomy, and new initiatives are often launched at the city level (Lieberthal 1995). Indeed the breathless pace of change in reform-era China has been characterized in part by incremental reforms pi-loted first in a select group of cities; the CDC system was first piloted in Shanghai (Peng et al. 2003). Many of the TM CDC's post-SARS reforms—the building of high-tech laboratories, the hiring of highly educated scien-tists, the coordination of local outbreak surveillance networks—were steps that were piloted in Tianmai and a few other cities with the idea that local CDCs around the country would eventually follow suit.

The "city of immigrants" model that Tianmai exemplifies also has been adopted around the country, as hundreds of millions of migrants flood cities from Beijing to Chongqing in search of a better life. China, as many scholars have noted, is "on the move" (Fong and Murphy 2006; Fan 2008). Living out one's life in one's hometown alongside parents or parents-in-law is no longer the norm but the exception (Ikels 2004). The busy, mobile, cosmopolitan lifestyle in Tianmai is becoming the norm all over China. Tianmai thus stands at the vanguard of China's future. That said, like all ethnographies, this study is a "view from somewhere" (Spencer 2001).

Global Health, Local Health

The view from somewhere that I present here offers a novel approach to the ethnographic study of global health. In focusing on a local government system in the most powerful non-Western country in the world as a critical node in a global network of disease control, this book decenters the dichotomous relationship between powerful Western actors and victimized non-Western locals presented in much of the ethnographic literature on global health (cf. Kim et al. 2002; Farmer 2003; Nichter 2008). Tianmai's public health professionals are neither victims nor power brokers; they are local but are part of the state; they are non-Western, but they aspire in some ways to be included in the Western world. And they are helping to remake "global health."

Although the meaning of the term *global health* is still hotly debated among scholars (Koplan et al. 2009; Fried et al. 2010; Crane 2013), anthropologists have disproportionately focused on the concept as it applies to humanitarian interventions and health-related aid. In particular, scholars have critiqued the often ill-fated efforts of powerful Western states like the United States— along with the NGOs and philanthropists who call these states home—to provide resources, training, and care to sick people residing in so-called weak states (Biehl and Petryna 2013; Farmer et al. 2013). The work that my informants did was not "global health" in this sense. China is nothing if not a strong state—and Tianmai was neither poor enough nor reliant enough on foreign assistance to fit in with this imaginary of global health.

Another definition of *global health*, as a term to describe the practice of global biosecurity, fits the Tianmai case more closely—but has received less ethnographic attention (for some exceptions, see Lakoff and Collier 2008; Lockerbie and Herring 2009; and Caduff 2014). If we take this second definition of global health-as-biosecurity as our jumping-off point, however, then in some ways the Chinese case stands out even more. SARS has widely been hailed as a wake-up call for Chinese biosecurity—a reminder to the Chinese state that it cannot and should not prioritize economic development over controlling dangerous diseases because if it does it is likely to achieve neither good health nor a persistently strong economy (cf. Kleinman and Watson 2006). And yet the Chinese state had already largely come to this conclusion itself before SARS arrived. SARS ultimately functioned, then, to provide not so much a threat or a push but an opportunity. The attention that the epidemic drew to biosecurity needs presented a way for a fledgling profession to rapidly gain clout and power for the first time in thirty years, provided a framework for how the CDCs should develop, and provided a platform from which to establish China as a scientifically sophisticated and even generous power on the global health stage. China's substantial technological, monetary, and human resources contributions to combating the Ebola epidemic in West Africa in late 2014 reflected this greater involvement as a global health power player: Having trained in one area of global health (biosecurity), the country was able to take the lead in another area of global health (humanitarian) as a provider, rather than a recipient, of aid (see Tiezzi 2014; UNDP 2014).

Ultimately, however, this is not a story about the global maneuverings of the central Chinese state. Instead, this book draws attention to the oft-neglected space between the nation-state and the people, opening a window into the opaque world of local Chinese governance. Understanding this interstitial space is critical to understanding how global health works in China and beyond.

Anthropologists have documented how powerful global health actors intervening in Africa or Latin America often sidestep, co-opt, or even ignore local governments as they mobilize their substantial resources to gain access to intervene on, and manipulate, local bodies. This results in negative unintended consequences for existing health infrastructure and services, as well as highly diminished, if not entirely absent, agency on the part of the state (Zaidi 1999; Benton 2015; Brown 2015), let alone the people whose bodies are being made available for study or intervention (Wendland 2012).

In contrast, in China foreign operators did *not* get to determine local public health agendas, and foreign actors were *not* able to easily gain access to local bodies. But the central government did not get to do these things either. Because of the decentralized nature of the Chinese state and strict rules on the operations of foreign individuals or organizations, local governments were the only entities that had access to local bodies. Thus any foreign actor who wished to do a health-related project at the local level was almost entirely dependent on the goodwill and cooperation of *local* public health professionals.

Because it was impossible for any foreign organization—even WHO or the U.S. CDC—to obtain permission to gain access to local people directly in China, foreign participation in public health programs in Tianmai was framed as a privilege rather than an act of charity. This sidestepped certain problems that came with excessive reliance on NGOs in other contexts, and allowed for a markedly different balance of power. As we will see in Chapters One and Three, however, it did little to protect local people's agency over their own bodies, which in China was simply claimed by local employers and local state agents rather than by foreign actors.

At the same time, influence over public health in China did sometimes flow along familiar geopolitical power gradients. My informants' foreign partners had a lot more power and influence than they admitted to or than the formal restrictions I just described would suggest. Chinese public health professionals' desire for acceptance into an idealized global health common, and more generally into a global common of modern global citizens, was a powerful force in allowing foreign influence to dominate and control even where it was technically not allowed to go. Eager to improve their own life chances, my interlocutors consciously attempted to orient their actions around what they perceived to be global norms and expectations. As a result, even the most mundane of their daily work often became deeply intertwined with the desires, needs, and oversight of actors that spanned the globe.

My informants' foreign collaborators were not at all unaware of the indirect influence they enjoyed—and yet their formal exclusion from the day-to-day management of Chinese populations provided some cover for what otherwise might be seen as, at best, questionably ethical actions on their part. Foreign researchers were able to obtain massive amounts of data via the hard work of ambitious Chinese collaborators who were willing to cut corners in obtaining consent (see Chapter Three), for example, and foreign governments were able to benefit from the involuntary surveillance and quarantines that local Chinese officials undertook on behalf of global pandemic prevention efforts (see Chapter Four). They did this by promoting a highly idealized vision of a better world and a better science that could result from these projects, seeding the dreams of a postsocialist populace thirsty for a new utopia.

Without any show of force or flood of NGO funding, American, European, and Australian global health scientists and practitioners thus were able to push forward their own agendas. And yet is precisely because China is *not* in an obviously vulnerable position, and because local governments there do *not* need foreign assistance in the way that those in other "global health" destinations do, that members of the global health community were so easily able to look the other way when ethical violations did occur. But this is a dangerous game. When foreign partners turn away from what is happening inside local spaces in China, they not only condone potential harm to individuals; they also aid and abet the bifurcation of service and governance.

The deep entanglement of global health and local public health that the Tianmai case draws out suggests one more important meaning embedded in "global health." Fried and colleagues in a 2010 article in the *Lancet* insisted that "global health and public health are indistinguishable," and that "global health" was just "public health" on a global scale and with a global perspective. As this definition suggests, and as the Tianmai case shows, the use of the term *global* can obscure the fact that all "global health" necessarily must concern itself with local populations and that a global "common good" necessarily represents one step on a continuum that stretches back to the local.

In the spirit of Fried's definition, what I lay out in these pages is a challenge to think through the Tianmai case not just as a window into public and global health in China but also as a window into local public health around the globe. Although the Chinese context may be unique, the challenges for the public health profession that are outlined in these pages are not. The tendency to draw boundaries around oneself and one's communities, the tensions between personal ties and professional responsibilities, and the desire to use one's education to reach ideals are common to the striving middle class the world over. The division between public health and medicine and the disciplinary boundaries that members of any profession tend to carefully police also are not peculiar to China. The tendency to govern the powerless in service of the powerful and the lack of trust that can result is one that all governments must combat. And the question of what professional responsibility means when one's "client" is an aggregate is a question for public health professionals anywhere. Rather than representing an exotic case, then, I suggest that the professionalization of public health in China after SARS offers a critical frame for rethinking what can and should constitute an ethical public health profession anywhere.

Chapter Overview

Each chapter of this book will explore a different dimension of public health professionals' efforts to govern and to serve. In Chapter One, "City of Immigrants," I take a closer look at the immigrant city of Tianmai, showing how my informants—former migrants themselves—actively maintained boundaries between themselves and the floating population as they worked to serve a *civilized immigrant common* of modern urban subjects.

In Chapter Two, "Relationships, Trust, and Truths," I show how the power to implement any given public health initiative was located within the *guanxi* webs that my informants spun anew at the beginning of each project. I illustrate the rituals through which *guanxi* was created and maintained and then consider how post-SARS public health workers attempted to establish a *professional common* that they hoped would make these rituals obsolete. In Chapter Three, "Scientific Imaginaries," I explore the efforts of Chinese public health professionals to advance their careers through scientific research. Newly hired young people labored to produce the "quality" and "true" data that they hoped would give them a chance to "develop themselves" as members of a *transnational scientific common*, raising new questions about global research ethics in the process.

In Chapter Four, "Pandemic Betrayals," I provide an eyewitness account of the TM CDC's response to the 2009 H1N1 influenza pandemic. I examine how my informants drew on the lessons of SARS and their professionalization project to mount what they thought would be an internationally lauded response to H1N1. Instead, Tianmai's public health professionals found that their full admittance into a *global common* or a *global health common* remained elusive. Finally, in the Conclusion, I examine the ways in which some public health professionals in Tianmai were experimenting with alternative interpretations of public health that broadened the boundaries of the common. I end by considering the implications of this ethnography for the study of public health—both local and global—more broadly.

Chapter One

City of Immigrants

Like millions of others from all over China, public health professionals migrated to Tianmai throughout the 1980s, 1990s, and 2000s to pursue what residents called, in a purposefully American fashion, the "Tianmai dream" (*tianmai mengxiang*). Predating by several years the broader "China dream" (*zhongguo meng*) later popularized by current Chinese president Xi Jinping, the "Tianmai dream" was for my interlocutors a natural outgrowth of Tianmai's identity as a "city of immigrants"—a moniker that implied freedom, possibility, and openness. Many of those whom I met in Tianmai told me that they came to the city because they saw it as a beacon that would free them from the small, stifling world of *guanxi* obligations, family ties, and dead-end jobs that they felt awaited them in their hometowns. Several also told me that they came because Tianmai was less "*paiwai*" (excluding of outsiders) than other big Chinese cities with similar opportunities, such as Guangzhou, Shanghai, and Beijing. My non-Cantonese informants in particular found this diverse enclave in the middle of Cantonese-dominated Guangdong province to be a breath of fresh air in a context in which they otherwise felt excluded linguistically and culturally. Yet after settling into their new homes and new jobs, most of the public health professionals I knew then went on to exclude the majority of their fellow migrants from this Tianmai dream.

In this chapter I argue that in their attempts to serve a *civilized immigrant common* emblematic of the Tianmai dream—as well as to protect their own preferred identities as privileged members of this common—Tianmai's public health professionals built and maintained precarious spatial, legal, historical, biological, moral, and professional boundaries between themselves and the 12 million strong floating population (*liudong renkou*) of rural-to-urban migrant workers that dominated the city. In building these boundaries, they established the majority of the residents of Tianmai as a population that had to be governed—but one that would not and could not be a part of a common to be served.[1]

The floating population and the civilized immigrant common reflected two sides of my interlocutors' "divided selves" (Kleinman et al. 2011). On one side was their past as members of poor peasant or worker families who toiled and suffered under a backward Maoist regime: the "population." On the other side was their future, as educated, cosmopolitan immigrants, living in a modern city that was uniquely free of the ghosts of a Maoist past: the "common." In this way, the migration of poor, rural people into the pristine modern city of Tianmai reflected a lingering fear on the part of that city's public health professionals that the side of their divided selves that they had left behind in the countryside would threaten the side that they had come to Tianmai to embrace.

The Floating Population

As of 2010, of Tianmai's estimated 16 million residents, 60 to 80 percent were categorized as *floating*—a term that describes the continuous movement of rural migrant workers from job to job and from the countryside to the city and back again.[2] According to C. Cindy Fan (2008), as of 2006, official estimates of China's floating population totaled about 150 million people nationwide. Informal estimates that my informants gave me in 2014 put the number somewhere closer to 250 million and growing. Rural villagers fled the Chinese countryside in the 1990s and 2000s, drawn to the cities by factory jobs and a chance to take part in the economic reforms that followed Mao's death. Legal residency requirements, however, prevented most of them from settling down permanently. As holders of rural household registrations (*hukou*), rural migrants living in cities continued to be tethered to their hometowns.

The central Chinese government established the *hukou* system of household registration in the 1950s as a means of monitoring and controlling population mobility between the countryside and the cities. All citizens were assigned at birth either rural or urban *hukou* status and generally were eligible for only the welfare and social services provided in their hometowns. This meant that a large majority of Chinese people was systematically excluded from many of the benefits associated with urban citizenship, including health care (Chan and Zhang 1999; Solinger 1999).

Governments at the central and local levels relaxed *hukou* restrictions with the start of the reforms in the early 1980s and continued to modify the law to be more permissive in the decades that followed. Nevertheless, in the late 2000s urban *hukou*s remained difficult to obtain—especially in the big cities and especially if one was not highly educated—and many rural residents who migrated to the cities remained excluded from the cities' benefits. Those who migrated to Tianmai without a *hukou* could apply for temporary or permanent "residence cards" that would qualify them for some of the benefits of urban registration, but migrants could get these only after going through extensive paperwork, meeting strict eligibility requirements, enduring long waiting periods, and often paying high fees.[3] In addition, as Li Zhang (2001) has described, many migrants feared that they would be found out by birth control authorities and fined for violating the one-child policy if they attempted to register. As a result, despite official assertions that the residency system accounted for all migrants, much of the floating population remained unaccounted for. Although they made up the backbone of Tianmai's economy and the majority of its population, a large proportion of migrants were officially not there.[4] And even where recent legal reforms began guaranteeing certain basic benefits for the migrants, laws were rarely enforced. For example, the state began granting certain limited legal rights to pensions (in 2006), health insurance (in 2008), and unemployment insurance (in 2013) to rural-to-urban migrants in the 2000s, but access and utilization remained quite limited (Mou et al. 2009; Lam and Johnston 2012; Magnier 2014).

One of the many implications of the *hukou* system was that Tianmai's public health professionals did not have to concern themselves as much as they otherwise might have with the mundane health concerns of its residents and in particular with the rising rates of chronic illness that were weighing down other health systems in urban China (He et al. 2005; Yang et al. 2008). Dr. Mi, a virologist, explained it to me this way: "Tianmai is a particular case because we depend on the *wailai renkou* [the outside population], but we don't take responsibility for their security. So if they get sick or old, or if they can't compete, they go home, and a new group of young people replaces them. So some people say that Tianmai exploits these young people. Actually, it is that way! Everyone gets old, but our burden for taking care of people who can't work anymore is small." As Pun Ngai (2005) has described, the transience of migrant labor was what the local Chinese state depended on, for in this way the state could extract labor from a population without having to take responsibility for the long-term well-being of the people who made up that population.

Though most major cities in China have significant floating populations, few are dominated by this population in quite the way Tianmai is. Shanghai and Beijing have large populations of migrants now, but they also are ancient cities with entrenched dominant local cultures. As Dorothy Solinger (1999) points out, Chinese internal migrants differ fundamentally from transnational migrants elsewhere in that "in this case the 'strangers' who were despised were China's own people" (4). Migrants in most Chinese cities, however, at least can still be categorized as out-of-place intruders, who by virtue of speaking a different dialect, eating a different cuisine, and having a different history, do not belong. Tianmai is different. Built just thirty-five years ago on land previously inhabited by only 30,000 people, there are very few people living in Tianmai today who are *not* migrants.

Tianmai thus has great ambivalence toward migration. Many of the TM CDC members I knew, like the migrants who made up the floating population, originally came from the countryside. But in informal conversations and interviews, public health professionals differentiated between "immigrants" (*yimin*), white-collar workers like themselves who had settled in Tianmai permanently and enjoyed legal and moral personhood, and migrants, sometimes referred to as "peasant workers" (*nongmingong*), or just peasants (*nongmin*), but usually simply grouped together as the "floating population" (*liudong renkou*). In calling Tianmai a "city of immigrants," my interlocutors compared it to the United States in a way that implied a forward-thinking, modern, creative society that attracted the best and brightest and offered freedoms not found elsewhere in China. The members of the floating population, being the wrong kinds of migrants, were not part of this immigrant dream.[5]

"Immigrants" made up the *civilized immigrant common* to be served. The "floating population," on the other hand, made up the *backward migrant population* to be governed. The use of the term *population* (*renkou*) in describing the floating migrants was important. As we saw in the Introduction, *renkou* in China is a statistical entity representative of a collective biology that needs to be tamed; it is the classic Foucauldian biopolitical object (Greenhalgh and Winckler 2005). For Tianmai's public health professionals, *renkou*, and especially *liudong renkou*, like the "masses" of Mao's time, functioned only as an undifferentiated aggregate. Public health professionals highlighted the undifferentiated nature of the floating population by speaking often of its high level of internal interchangeability. My informants told me that it was usually useless to try to reach this population with health messages that might benefit it, for example, because if one person was reached that person would soon be replaced by another—leaving the population as a whole unchanged and maddeningly incapable of internalizing healthy change. Dr. Mi explained, "If you go there and try to educate them, say about HIV, then a few days later they all switch . . . and you have to start over." Mi's effort to serve the floating population ran up against the constraints of a mobile existence. He told me that many of his colleagues reasoned that urban public health professionals should not even make the kinds of outreach attempts that Mi did, both because they would inevitably fail and also because when members of the floating population got sick or their health deteriorated in old age they would—and should—just "go home" (*huijia*) to their rural villages.

The assumption that rural migrants would eventually just "go home" bolstered the case for my interlocutors that the floating population could not become part of a civilized immigrant common. Another assumption that bolstered this case was the association that public health professionals made between migrants' mobility and their assumed filth. To migrate is to breach boundaries; thus all migrants are, in Mary Douglas's (2002) sense at least, unclean. Indeed the trope of migrants as dirty has stubbornly persisted over time and in a wide range of local contexts (Markel 1997; Shah 2001; Molina 2006; Horton and Barker 2009). But while Tianmai's public health professionals cleansed themselves of the countryside by building new lives as urban citizens, on arriving in the city the floating population failed to do the same, instead constantly recrossing boundaries from city to countryside and job to job. In continually rebreaching the boundaries between rural and urban, these new migrants made it impossible to "rid [themselves] of the contamination of their 'feudal' past" (Anagnost 1997, 11). Dr. Ying, a parasitologist at one of the district CDCs told me in an interview:

> The countryside in China is very dirty, very chaotic, very inferior [*cha*]. This is true in some parts of Tianmai too—have you been to the chaotic parts of Tianmai? . . . [These places] are even more serious [than the countryside]. Why? Because where people live, it's not their own home, they are renting, they don't plan to stay for a long time, so they don't care about keeping it clean, they figure they will be leaving soon, so why bother? So it is filthy.

Dr. Ying, who himself grew up in a fishing village in rural eastern Guangdong, saw the peasants who littered his pristine modern city as an unwelcome reminder of his own rural past and a contaminating presence in the new life he had tried to build for himself.

Especially after the arrival of SARS, the floating population's supposed filth also became indicative of the risk of contagious disease spread. TM CDC members blamed the floating population for Tianmai's failure to eliminate certain diseases that they associated with backwardness, such as measles; for exposing the common to certain endemic diseases, such as hepatitis; and for threatening to incubate new diseases, such as H1N1 influenza. One informant noted, for example, that even after multiple vaccination campaigns, as of 2009 Tianmai had the highest measles rates in Guangdong province. With each attempt at citywide eradication, he complained to me, came a new wave of immune-deficient migrants from the countryside, who, he said, crowded into factories and tenement housing and spread the disease like wildfire.

In a kind of inversion of Adriana Petryna's notion of biological citizenship, the migrants' inferior biology thus established them as threats to the city that needed to be controlled, rather than as citizens of the city who needed to be helped. For Petryna (2002), biological citizenship in post-Chernobyl Ukraine was a means of gaining access to social services, whereby "the damaged biology of a population has become the grounds for social membership and the basis of staking citizenship claims" (5). In post-SARS Tianmai, the situation was just the opposite: The supposedly inferior biology of the floating population became grounds for a lack of social membership and for a denial, rather than a granting, of citizenship claims.

This is not a new story: In many ways, the biological noncitizenship of Tianmai's migrant population mirrors a situation common to immigrants throughout history, whereby allegations of poor hygiene and disease among immigrant groups often served as an excuse for exclusion and persecution and as a powerful mechanism for turning persons into biological threats (Markel 1997; Shah 2001; Briggs and Mantini-Briggs 2003; Molina 2006). The contemporary Tianmai case was peculiar in at least two respects, however: The group doing the excluding was itself made up almost entirely of migrants, often hailing from the same regions as those they were excluding, and the group being excluded was, on the surface, quite similar to the group that played an essential role in *eliminating* disease in China in the past.

Before their transformation into a "population" and their migration to the cities, rural peasants made up the bulk of the *qunzhong* ("masses")—that undifferentiated group of Communist foot soldiers that fueled Chairman Mao's public health campaigns. Although the masses were blamed for the spread of infectious disease even during Mao's time, they also served as the solution to their own problem. Their large numbers and ideological commitment meant that they could be made to participate in mass sanitation work and mass vaccinations (see Introduction). The floating population of today, however, posed a problem without offering a solution. Mao's methods could never be repeated in the present day, my informants told me: It would simply be too hard to locate people who were always in motion, and those people could not be counted on to comply with public health measures.

The inability to control the floating population created considerable anxiety for those charged with preventing another SARS-like event. Huang Qing, an epidemiologist who worked on infectious disease surveillance, told me in an interview during the 2009 H1N1 influenza outbreak:

> The floating population really terrifies me. [The migrants] are a really special problem here—everyone is terrified of them! (*xia si ren!*) Because there is no way to keep track of them, no one has any idea where they are, and if there is really a pandemic, then we're in big trouble! Their *wenhua* [cultural level] is low; a lot are from the countryside, they don't understand basic biological facts, and they don't have any responsibility, no sense of that at all, and so if we

come looking for them to check up if we think they have flu, they'll just think, "You're trying to do what?" and they'll run away to some other place and go find work there. And then we'll have no idea where they are—we can't keep track—we find this very scary! There is no way to maintain social stability in that situation.

Huang's comments suggest that the potential social instability associated with the floating population was at least as frightening as—and inseparable from—their potential contagiousness. As Ann Anagnost (1997) argues, "Although [the migrants'] cheap labor fuels the explosive expansion of the reform economy, their very presence raises the specter of social disorder and political instability. They are the uncivilized crowd that has not yet been made into a modern citizenry, the unsightly but indispensable presence in the heart of China's civility" (136). In 2008, when the global financial crisis prompted hundreds of Tianmai's factories to close down and many thousands of migrants to suddenly lose their jobs, several informants told me that what they most feared was what might happen if this uncivilized crowd suddenly ceased to be indispensable. One TM CDC worker noted, "When people are not employed, things get chaotic."

Fear of chaos and social instability has been a persistent theme in reform-era China, fueled by memories of suffering endured during the Great Leap Forward and the Cultural Revolution.[6] Erica James (2008), following Anthony Giddens, describes a sense in Haiti of "ontological insecurity," where "there is no presumption of stability, security or trust for the individual or collective group" (138). A version of this ontological insecurity created during the chaotic Mao years persisted for many in reform-era China—especially among those who remembered the previous era clearly and knew all too well how quickly the tide could turn against them. After recounting her own childhood living through the latter years of the Cultural Revolution and her later rise through the ranks of China's educated middle class, Huang told me, for example: "I don't think I'll be here [in China] forever. Because I already want to give myself an escape route. It is the wisdom of Chinese people to take precautions for self-protection. . . . I mean that you have to give yourself another option. This is the only way you won't risk ending up in a miserable situation like my mother's parents, starving to death [in the Great Leap Forward]" (see also Osburg 2013). For Tianmai's public health professionals, the fears of instability that these memories evoked became intertwined with fears of disorder that the floating population represented. In doing their best to control this dangerous population, they were also doing their best to stabilize their own lives. The population that threatened the common was for them the past that threatened their future.

The Boundaries of Urban Space

Even as it became overwhelmingly dominant as a demographic force and a perceived social danger, much of the floating population in Tianmai managed to remain, to a surprising degree, invisible. At times this invisibility could be quite disorienting. For example, as we drove to a local hospital in the Tianmai subdistrict of Gongping for an inspection on an afternoon in the fall of 2008, Dr. Li, an epidemiologist at the TM CDC, told me that the conditions at the hospital would likely be quite good because "people who live in Gongping are really rich" (*zhu zai Gongping de ren dou hen youqian*)— they all lived in really nice gated communities (*xiaoqu*) and drove fancy cars. I was confused—hadn't he also told me that Gongping had a huge floating population? And wasn't the floating population poor? Dr. Li looked at me quizzically, before acknowledging that yes, 90 percent of the population was in fact floating, and this population was in fact poor. But that was not what he meant when he referred to "people who live in Gongping."[7]

One of the things that made it possible to keep such a dominant presence invisible in the urban environment is that most rural migrants lived in spaces in the city that were not entirely urban to begin with, congregating in factory dormitories or cheap apartment blocks inside Tianmai's "villages-in-the-city" (*chengzhongcun*). Tianmai residents love to tell visitors that thirty years ago their booming metropolis was a small "fishing village." But the mythology of the fishing village-to-city transition is belied by the fact that Tianmai was built not of one village, but of hundreds, and that these villages continue to play an important role in the city's governance (see O'Donnell 2001; Bach 2010).

The villages that became Tianmai all were officially urbanized by 2004, yet they remained relatively autonomous entities, subject to only limited city controls. When Tianmai was first established as an urban unit in 1980, the communized village land incorporated into the city initially was left with rural status. Thus while the land *between* villages was urbanized, and while the villagers eventually were given urban residency status, the villages themselves functioned as semiautonomous rural pockets that continued to be ruled by village leaders—many of whom became extremely wealthy as their land exploded in value. Because the villages were at first technically neither urban nor under the jurisdiction of the city government, and because they were subject to only limited city controls, village leaders found myriad ways to avoid adhering to official regulations limiting the types of buildings that could be built on their land, how many people could live there, or how services such as sanitation and security had to be managed (see Zhang 2001; Siu 2007; Bach 2010). Providing cheap housing in an otherwise expensive housing market and refuge from city institutions that sought to register and even deport migrant workers, the owners of the apartment blocks—the villagers of old—ended up acting as slumlords for the newly arrived migrants (Bach 2010).[8]

This state of affairs largely persisted even following waves of official village urbanization in the 1990s and 2000s, and it established geographical and spatial boundaries between settled migrants who lived outside of the villages and floating migrants who did not. The settled migrants built new middle-class lives in ultramodern high-rise buildings that fit easily into the cityscape. The floating population, on the other hand, remained in a state of what Cho calls "inclusive exclusion" (2013). They were included within the city limits yet seemed frozen in place within a crumbling rural environment, as the city continued to grow up around them. Living in slum conditions inside the villages contributed to the unclassifiability of floating population members, increased their vulnerability to disease while decreasing their access to services, and left public health professionals at the mercy of what they called a "feudal" village system when mounting disease control efforts. Living in the villages thus perpetuated migrants' biological noncitizenship through a vicious cycle: Their ghettoization in unregulated low-income housing communities increased their risk of disease, whereas their assumed riskiness justified further exclusion—all while making it difficult for public health professionals to reach them.[9]

To gain access to the floating population for a 2009 measles vaccination campaign, for example, my colleagues at the municipal level had to rely on *guanxi* connections with district- and street-level public health institutions to indirectly connect them to factory bosses and village leaders. As I will explore more in the next chapter, these sorts of *guanxi* negotiations were critical for accomplishing any public health project, but for projects necessitating access to the villages they were especially difficult to navigate because of the villages' highly independent leadership structures. Many of the Cantonese- and Hakka-speaking village leaders were openly defiant of Tianmai government mandates and contemptuous of the Mandarin-speaking teams that came in from city institutions.[10] Bringing village leaders on board thus necessitated intensive *guanxi* building with ambitious intermediate actors at the street-level CDCs who shared linguistic and cultural ties with the village leaders but who also harbored ambitions for moving up in the public health system in Tianmai. It was these street-level actors who were able to connect my city CDC colleagues to village leaders—but my informants were not necessarily able to secure cooperative intermediaries like these for every village in Tianmai.

Tianmai's public health professionals complained that village leaders had no regard for public health and no place in an urban setting. Health workers who worked within the villages also complained of this problem. When conducting a malaria-reporting compliance inspection at a dilapidated hospital in one village, for example, my colleagues shook their heads in disgust that such a "rich village" could have such poor compliance and such poor hospital conditions. The chastised hospital workers in turn complained that their poor compliance was because of their own "exploitation" by the "feudal" village boss, who refused to invest in hospital infrastructure or disease control systems and instead kept all of their money for himself. Ultimately, the taint of this "feudal" system fell on the entire village and its inhabitants. By remaining stubbornly backward while also housing the rural migrant workers that drove the modern city's rapid urban economic growth, the villages, and the floating population with them, served as "both a key locus for China's urban civilizing mission and the lump in its urban throat" (Bach 2010, 447).

Thanks to the floating population's association with chaos, this lump in the urban throat also represented urban danger. Floating migrants were the most likely to commit crimes, steal their wallets, or hurt them after dark, my TM CDC informants told me. I was told to stay away from urban villages and other areas where the floating population liked to congregate, especially at night. In this milieu, many public health professionals saw the space and community provided to them by the TM CDC *danwei* (work unit) as an oasis of safety. The *danwei* provided my interlocutors with exactly what many of their peers who had come to Tianmai to *xiahai*, or "jump into the sea of business," lacked: permanent employment, a stable, close-knit community, and a physical space where they could feel protected.

The *danwei* community was grounded in face-to-face interpersonal relationships and *guanxi* connections; It was the same kind of community that many had eagerly left behind in their own villages. Dr. Mi noted that "in our hometowns [we] knew all our neighbors but now [in Tianmai we] might not even know who lives next door." Within the confines of the TM CDC, however, everyone still knew everyone else. Although most *danwei* members no longer lived on the grounds of their work unit as they did during the Mao period, many employees lived in gated communities (*xiaoqu*) that were at least partially subsidized by the TM CDC and that housed mainly employees in their own or related *danweis*. Young unmarried people tended to live together with peers from the *danwei* and eventually married within the *danwei* or within the larger public health system of associated *danweis*. They mostly restricted socializing to fellow *danwei* members or university classmates. They did not easily trust outsiders.

The TM CDC was relatively homogenous compared with many *xiaoqus* and especially with the city as a whole. Most members hailed from a few distinct parts of China—certain areas of Hunan and Sichuan provinces and the Guangzhou and Chaozhou regions in Guangdong—and were educated at a small handful of South Chinese medical colleges. School allegiances ran deep, particularly among those who attended the same medical college as the CDC director. Not only was Director Lan more likely to hire students and graduates of his alma mater, he and the other leaders also often granted favors based on school allegiance.

Thus, even as Tianmai's public health professionals embraced the romance of the city of immigrants, their everyday lives were deeply entrenched in a traditional community structure established by the bounds of their *danwei* and its internal *guanxi* networks. This allowed them to explore the immigrant city from a familiar home base. Though they glamorized the freedom that Tianmai was supposed to represent—freedom from the *guanxi*-based sociality of their hometowns, proximity to a quasi-international border, a diversity of people and opportunities—my interlocutors also told me that they were relieved to have the *danwei*, quintessential bastion of Communist urban social organization, as an anchor of stability.[11]

For TM CDC members, Tianmai became divided into two classes of people: "*women danwei de*" (of our *danwei*) and "*bushi women danwei de* (not of our *danwei*). Among those with whom one did not have another type of personal connection, generally only those "of our *danwei*" could be trusted. TM CDC members repeatedly urged me, as an honorary member of the *danwei*, to find roommates and friends only within the *danwei* or among "friends" of *danwei* members—outside of these circles I could never be certain what threats might lurk. This, then, was the hardest boundary that my informants drew between themselves and the floating population: The floating population was most certainly "not of our *danwei*."[12]

As Li Zhang (2010) has described in the case of Kunming City, members of Tianmai's privileged classes who were not affiliated with government institutions like the TM CDC also independently sought out some of the urban cloistering that the *danwei* facilitated by purchasing homes in *xiaoqus*. Zhang (2010) and Tomba (2014) describe how buying a home within a *xiaoqu* has become a cornerstone of the Chinese middle-class dream. These gated communities create a geographic and spatial reality around the symbolic and legal exclusion of unpredictable outside populations, form isolated pockets of increased social trust, and allow for what Zhang calls "governing through community"—a form of governmentality in which semiautonomous *xiaoqus* provide many of governing functions of the state that also were previously delegated to *danweis*.

With its dozens or even hundreds of urban villages, *xiaoqus*, and *danweis*, the segmented spatial and political geography of Tianmai both perpetuated boundaries between worthy and unworthy immigrants and also further detached public health from local spaces. In the Introduction I noted that the goals of public health in previous periods had been explicitly spatial and proximate: Maintaining a clean local space was the number one priority of local public health institutions. But with local spaces so divided in Tianmai, the city and district CDCs had little ability or motivation to keep every piece of the fragmented cityscape clean and healthy. The city's segmentation thus fueled the bifurcation of service and governance. Tianmai's public health professionals sought to vaccinate, test, and study the floating population wherever they were able to gain access to it, in the hopes that the civilized immigrant common—the group they imagined resided in all the clean and sparkly *xiaoqus* of the city—could protect its safe and healthy way of life.

The Hukou *System*

As spatially segmented as Tianmai was, the floating population could and did often traverse these spatial boundaries. But one of the most stubborn and most difficult boundaries to cross remained a legal one: the boundary between *hukou*-carrying immigrants and non–*hukou*-carrying migrants. Though my interlocutors were not responsible for creating this boundary, very few were eager to dismantle it. In supporting the usefulness and rightness of the *hukou* policy, Tianmai's public health professionals increased the policy's power and contributed to the legal separation of worthy and unworthy migrants.

Those who were lucky enough to have obtained a Tianmai *hukou* after being born into a rural one—generally by virtue of their early migration, their association with a *danwei* like the TM CDC, their high level of education, or their use of *guanxi* connections (or all of the above)—often expressed discomfort with the idea of extending this privilege to the floating population. Some worried that doing so might threaten their own social positions and spark greater social instability. For example, several of my interlocutors defended the government-mandated rules in Tianmai and other cities whereby floating migrants diagnosed with HIV were denied the free antiretroviral drugs guaranteed under China's "Four Frees and One Care" program because, in keeping with the *hukou* system, "It is the responsibility of their hometowns to give it to them."[13] They readily admitted that most floating migrants could not realistically return to their villages for treatment because they would lose their jobs and be subject to intense stigma at home. Yet several interlocutors insisted that, regrettably, this policy of biological noncitizenship was necessary to "uphold order" in Tianmai. If they made drugs available to all migrants, these public health professionals asserted, then there would be an uncontrollable flood of HIV-positive populations from all over China who would descend on Tianmai to obtain free services.[14] Their implication was that these dirty populations, in addition to spreading instability and creating economic strain, would then spread HIV to *hukou*-carrying persons (Hyde 2007).

A lack of access to urban privileges like health care, however, was one of the factors that kept the floating migrants in motion and perpetuated the instability of the population (see Willen 2007; Goldade 2009). The Tianmai government repeatedly declared its commitment to addressing this problem and in 2006 launched the "Medical Insurance System for Migrant Employees" (MISM), which legally required large employers to register their migrant employees for a special basic health insurance scheme; a similar scheme for migrant children was launched in 2008 (Lam and Johnston 2012; Mou et al. 2013). A 2009 study of this project found that employers failed to add most migrants to the scheme, tending to offer the services only to their least mobile, most highly skilled workers (Mou et al. 2009). By 2011, 5.3 million migrants were technically covered by the program, though a 2012 study found continued low registration rates (Lam and Johnston 2012; Mou et al. 2013). Those who did enroll in the program used services only slightly more than those who did not—probably, several informants told me, because they were afraid that if they went to a hospital their illegal status would be discovered.[15]

Dr. Mi told me that although efforts to provide more services for migrants were noble, he doubted that greater access to health care would solve the floating population problem. A deeper source for the persistent infectiousness of migrants, he told me, came from an ethical failing on the part of the migrants themselves. In explaining why migrant workers had high rates of HIV/AIDS, for example, he explained, "The problem is that they leave their families, and then their sense of responsibility is gone. See, if they were around relatives and close friends, then they would fear getting a bad reputation, so they wouldn't do immoral things. Like those of us with family here, we don't want to cause problems for our family, so we won't do bad things." If the migrants would only put down roots and build the kinds of kin and *guanxi* networks that those in his *danwei* enjoyed, they too could become responsible, full-fledged citizens of Tianmai. And yet Mi's argument was also circular: It is precisely because they were *not* treated as Tianmai citizens that the floating migrants did not stay in the city and form those relationships. As Saskia Sassen (2006) has suggested, without the right to fully integrate into the city, the floating migrants lacked the moral status to demand that this right be granted.

Heroic Migrants and the Great Malaria Epidemics

The imaginary of the rural-to-urban migrant to Tianmai was not always so negative. In fact, if one looks to the other side of the historical boundary that some of Tianmai's earliest immigrants drew between themselves and the floating population, one can see that migrants of a different sort were the mythic heroes of Tianmai's early days. It was migrants, after all, who came in the 1970s and 1980s to transform the villages into a new city by constructing Tianmai's first roads, buildings, and power plants. A plaque in Tianmai's city history museum declared that, when Tianmai was established,

> The Central Military Commission deployed over 20,000 military construction engineers to support the construction of [Tianmai]. Constructors from all over the country came to [Tianmai], as the "trailblazing ox" (*kaihuang niu*). Through several years of hard work, the urban infrastructure construction of [Tianmai] began to take shape. [Tianmai] was called a "City That Rose Overnight" (*yiye cheng*) and created the ["Tianmai speed"] known all over the country.

Above this inscription was a grainy photograph of smiling workers laying railroad tracks. As the inscription suggested, these first migrants were celebrated as both literal and figurative "trailblazers" who converted Tianmai overnight from a backward rural place into an urban paradise. Included among these trailblazers was a small group of public health workers.

In the 1980s and early 1990s malaria epidemics ravaged the fledgling city of Tianmai and threatened to swallow it up in its rural underpinnings. These epidemics also brought much of the older generation of public health workers to Tianmai. Although migrants to Tianmai in the twenty-first century brought contamination and backwardness to a modern city, my interlocutors told me, the public health professionals who migrated to Tianmai during the 1980s brought health and civilization to a rural backwater.

As with many other civilizing and colonizing projects, the founding of Tianmai was fraught with biological assaults. Like the builders of the Panama Canal who met early deaths at the hands of yellow fever and the European colonizers of Africa who succumbed to other diseases, malaria overwhelmed the first arrivals to Tianmai, which was then a wet, humid marsh. This was a detail left out of the romanticized version of Tianmai's history presented in the museum, but it was this aspect that my older informants remembered the best because it was malaria, they told me, that secured them a place in building the Tianmai dream. Most remembered this period fondly, even when recounting the hardships involved.

A fifty-five-year-old TM CDC member who arrived with the first cohort of public health workers dispatched to Tianmai told me that after graduating from vocational high school (*zhongzhuan*) she worked in the poor rural province of Guangxi for ten years:

But in the early 1980s when Tianmai was first being developed, I heard they were looking for people to control a major malaria epidemic that was killing off the people who were coming here to build; they wanted people who already had experience, so I took the opportunity and came. Environment-wise, Guangxi was better—Tianmai was very *luan* [chaotic]—everyone was building and building; it was a big mess. There was nowhere really to live or eat, very isolated . . .

We had controlled [malaria] by 1988–1989, then it came back in 1992–1993. . . . The second time we controlled it was 1995–1996, but at that point living standards were really rising, it was really developed here, *suzhi* [quality of people] was higher, and we could control it for good. Because it used to be rural, Tianmai had fields and things, but then it became a city, and there was nowhere for the mosquitoes to breed.

In a speech at a TM CDC event, another middle-aged woman recounted:

I came from Yunnan, and it was pretty backward, but you can't imagine how poor and backward it was in Tianmai, much worse than Yunnan—in Yunnan we had thatched mud brick cottages—here we just had work sheds—we couldn't even do the [DDT] spraying properly; the sheds didn't have walls to spray onto. One by one the workmen were falling. The city government told us, you have one year to control it, three to eradicate. Everyone had to pitch in, soaking bed nets and spraying. We used a really strong DDT spray back then, and we had no protective gear and had to soak so many bed nets per year; it was a slow process. We rubbed our fingers raw, and the chemicals corroded our skin, and we had allergic reactions. Our fingers were rubbed raw, and when we walked our feet were drenched in blood.

Then there was the survey to measure how many mosquitoes there were. Every ten days there was a day where for fifteen minutes every hour we counted mosquitoes. We stood between the cow and human sheds and sometimes our feet were deep in cow dung; the stench was unbearable. Also the mosquitoes could get us if our gear was not tight, and we could smell the sweet smell of mosquitoes having just eaten, along with the cow dung. We did this all night until morning. Once our team leader contracted malaria, but he took medicine and kept going; we were all very moved by this.

The hardships that they endured on their arrival became a key part of the lure of Tianmai's history for public health professionals: Tianmai was able to develop into a modern city by driving out a backward disease through the grit and hard work of dedicated public health workers.

Even those public health professionals who had not participated in the campaigns celebrated the perseverance of those who, toughened by their own rural pasts, had not been afraid to suffer. Explaining that the malaria veterans had retained the peasant virtue of "the ability to 'eat bitterness' (*chi ku*) or endure hardship" (Jacka 2006, 53), Dr. Pu, a forty-year-old man who works on malaria today, told me:

> You look at how successful we were with malaria—even Singapore still has malaria, and look at how modern and sanitary they are. So how come we could get rid of it here and they didn't there? It's because we are willing to suffer and stick with it, and persevere—the West talks so much about "human rights," but we have a collectivist spirit (*jitizhuyi jingshen*). And even several years ago, when our country was very poor, we still did it [won against malaria] to the level that we did. So this is something very special about us.

In Pu's view, Tianmai was protected through the collectivist ethic of its settlers and their willingness to sacrifice themselves for a cause. Pu was unusual among the younger cohort of TM CDC employees in his reverence for Communist values, but older members of the TM CDC in their fifties and sixties very often took pride in their history of fortitude and their commitment to collectivist values. Said one older interlocutor:

> Back then everyone was poor, costs were low, and *sixiang* [ideas] were really different; demands were low, there weren't material demands like now after the reforms. Now society has advanced, but people chase material things a lot more . . . Back then it was the *jingshen* [spirit, energy] factor. There was more *jingshen*. Back then the barefoot doctors' earnings were very small. But now it would take a lot more investment [to do something like that].

At the same time, even the older members of the TM CDC did not celebrate the role of the untrained masses in their stories—the heroes of the campaigns of Mao's day (see Introduction). Instead, even as they told their stories of sacrifice, they also emphasized the critical importance of their own expertise and education. They were never exactly backward peasants themselves, despite their modest upbringings, they explained—they always had stood out as educated people with the ability to become civilized and urban. The man quoted above extolling China's "collectivist spirit," for example, also argued that the victory over malaria only happened through the perseverance of trained workers. And only the "experts" who had been brought in since SARS could tackle an epidemic like malaria if it happened again:

> Then SARS happened, and the government paid attention again . . . and then they realized that just because you don't have a disease like malaria now doesn't mean it won't appear in the future. So you want to have these people around. These experts who would know what to do should it appear again—you have people coming over from Africa, returning from travel, and if you have no malaria people, no department, then who's going to deal with it? And then it will spread.

References to far-flung travel as a source of disease also pointed to the multitude of ways in which the heightened mobility of the Chinese people seemed poised to topple the very modernity that made such mobility possible. It was not only migrants who were dangerous: Tourists and wealthy Chinese travelers had the potential to bring contamination back to Tianmai as well. During the course of my fieldwork, for example, a parasite found primarily in husky dogs in Tibet began appearing among businesspeople in Tianmai; the culprit was a pet dog purchased during a family vacation to Lhasa. Under these circumstances the wealthy, too, could become *renkou*: When I returned to Tianmai for follow-up fieldwork in 2014, *fuyou renkou*, or the "wealthy population," had become a growing target of concern, referring primarily to those nouveaux riches who engaged in irresponsible and excessive acts like buying Tibetan dogs or overindulging in fatty foods. The mobility of wealthy residents and visitors, and the potential for them, too, to carry diseases, rendered the line between "good" and "bad" migrants all the more precarious.

Managing Migrant Bodies

The precarious line between good and bad migrants required a great deal of maintenance—especially when the two kinds of migrants came directly into contact with each other. Most public health professionals in Tianmai dealt with the floating population only in the abstract, through the design of interventions carried out by anonymous others connected to them through a series of *guanxi* relationships and through the compilation of the statistics that were produced as a result. However, those who worked in the outpatient clinics at the local CDCs—where a steady stream of migrants came to undergo the physical exams (*tijian*) necessary to obtain a "health license" (*jiankang zheng*) to work in service businesses—had daily contact with migrants. The physicals served a dual purpose: They ensured that migrants working legally were free of infectious diseases, and they also provided an important source of cash flow for the CDC system.[16] At the same time, they established moral boundaries between "high-" and "low-quality" (*suzhi*) migrants.

To be assigned to an outpatient clinic team was a fate that many public health professionals, both young and old, regarded as degrading. "The problem is that there are just so many of them, and their *suzhi* [quality] is just so low," said one clinic worker with a master's degree in molecular epidemiology. "It's also so boring, and such a waste of my education." The descriptions that several informants gave of their interactions with the migrants during the physical exams were especially notable for their expressions of disgust—disgust that was evocative of reactions to racially marked people and immigrants in other contexts (Mason 2015). As a TM CDC member in her late thirties told me of her time several years earlier working on a clinic team,

> Four or five days a week I had to go to the factory and do physicals on the workers. And it was horrible! It was so hot and stuffy that I felt as if I was going to die! And all the workers were dirty and all sweaty; there was so much sweat! And their skin had all these problems, and you had to touch them to do the exam—it was disgusting, and it felt very unsafe there, it was so hot and sweaty. When I came back, I would feel so dirty. And we would sometimes go through 1,000 people in one day. . . . I couldn't take it—I got myself transferred as soon as I could.

For two weeks I volunteered in an outpatient clinic at one of the district-level CDCs and also went with several mobile teams to a sauna, a restaurant, and an entertainment center. I quickly began to understand why my informants reacted to the migrant patients in the way that they did. In the clinic I swabbed fingers, numbered forms, and pushed lines along. In the long hours on this assembly line of endless bodies that had to be processed, I too felt an overwhelming sense of visceral distaste. I was hot, the oxygen felt drained from the room, the people seemed slow and uncooperative, the stench of hundreds of people's body odors filled my nose, the line of bodies wound around and around seemingly without end, and I found myself feeling angry, frustrated, annoyed, bitter at those bodies that would not stop coming, those fingers that had to be swabbed one by one, without a break, every ten seconds. In this environment, it was difficult to see the migrants as persons in need of care; for those two weeks, their significance for me, as for many of my interlocutors, was as biological matter that had to be processed as quickly as possible. The clinical encounter transformed the floating population from a statistical entity into a collection of biological bodies, but it was an encounter entirely lacking in intersubjective engagement. Whereas the public health professionals felt disgust, the embodied experiences of the migrants themselves were irrelevant to my informants, who rarely acknowledged the possibility of their clients' discomfort (Buch 2013). (See Figure 1.1.)

A typical worker on the physical exam line saw 600 to 1,000 patients in a day, the large majority of them members of the floating population. Workers took sanitary precautions more to protect themselves than to protect the patients: Workers did not change gloves between patients, for example, and they left needles and cotton swabs out in the open uncovered. At one point I knocked over a rack of needles, and the nurse who was training me picked them up from the floor by hand, replaced them in the rack, and used them for the next round of patients. On the other hand, when I handed out forms to the patients, the nurses chided me for not wearing gloves, incredulous that I was willing to take the chance of touching one of the workers' hands as I handed them the forms.

Patients first paid a fee at a cashier's counter, had their photos taken, were given a form and a number, and then were sent to an assembly line at a long open table to have their fingers swabbed with alcohol and then pricked for blood. At the end of the line each patient was handed a large red syringelike tube and sent to one of two open rooms, segregated by sex. Migrants waiting

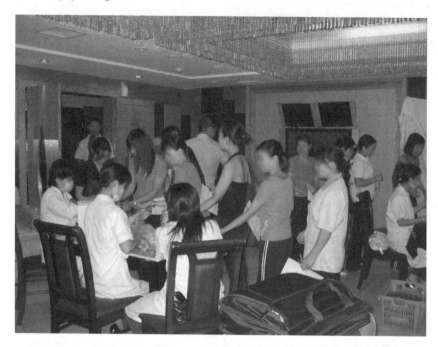

Figure 1.1. A traveling migrant clinic run by one of Tianmai's district CDCs visits an entertainment venue to conduct physical exams, 2008.
Photo by the author.

their turn crowded in, peering over each other's heads. On the female side, a harried worker barked at each migrant in turn to bend over and pull down her pants; she inserted the red tube in the migrant's anus, put the tube in a rack, and barked for the next person to come forward and bend over. The fecal sample was used to look for common intestinal bacterial diseases.

After the fecal sample was taken, the migrants were sent on to an X-ray room, where they marched in one by one to have their lungs examined. Each patient stood in the room for several seconds while the technician examined the lungs for signs of tuberculosis; no lead protection was offered. Following the X-ray, the exam was over; beyond pricking fingers, the examiners never touched the patients. Although factories conducted somewhat more involved exams (where conditions such as hearing loss were tested), "Our goal is to make sure these people are not spreading diseases to the general population through their services, especially those that involve food," one clinic worker told me. After the exam, the patient received a receipt and instructions to come back in a few days to get the results. Often an employer representative was given a stack of receipts for 100 or more migrants and told to pick up all of the results him- or herself. The employer thus managed knowledge about migrant bodies and shared this knowledge with the individual at his or her own discretion.

For the two weeks in which I volunteered in the clinic, I became part of the establishment conducting the tests. This had at least two important implications: First, I became involved in a process that I found ethically problematic in its utilization of, and demeaning attitude toward, migrant bodies. This raised ethical questions, with which I struggled throughout my fieldwork, about the acceptability of contributing to this exercise in my role as participant-observer. Second, it was impossible for me to have any meaningful conversations with the migrants themselves about this process. This was not my project—others (Zhang 2001; Murphy 2002; Ngai 2005; Jacka 2006) have devoted years to studying how rural-to-urban migrants in China live, what they think, and how they embody their oppression. Nevertheless, I did spend two days conversing with migrant workers in the settings where they were being screened, during which time I was able to discern that few had any idea what they were being tested for. Several gave an embarrassed "I'm not sure" to my questions; some were able to name TB and hepatitis as diseases for which they were tested; no one had any idea what the fecal samples were for. When I mentioned this to one of the clinic workers, she shook her head: "I tried to tell you, it's no use trying to talk to them. Their *suzhi* [quality] is too low, and they have no idea what you're asking, they don't understand even the most basic things. . . . If you want to know something about them, it's better to ask their boss."

The assumption that ignorance and incompetence on the part of the migrant workers lay behind migrant behaviors—as opposed to poor communication on the part of the clinic workers—was ubiquitous.[17] When I suggested to one clinic worker that instead of screening all food workers for certain diseases they could simply encourage them to wear gloves, the horrified worker told me, "Oh no, maybe that would work in your country, where people have higher *suzhi*, but these people could not be trusted to wear gloves!"

Suzhi in reform-era China was associated with personhood (Fong 2007), with subjectivity (Ong 2006), and with an ability to take on the responsibilities of modern neoliberal citizenship (see Jacka 2006). Having *suzhi* meant one could act as a fully integrated person in society by participating actively in one's own health regulation. This was accomplished through asking and answering questions, understanding instructions, and caring for one's body. Lacking *suzhi* meant that one was not a fully agentive person, could not be trusted to understand or carry out any bodily maintenance on one's own, and needed instead to be carefully controlled.

The clinic worker linked the inability of migrants to take measures to restrict their own infectiousness to their low *suzhi*. In keeping with neoliberal assumptions about the need for self-regulation in the promotion of health, many of the public health professionals I knew felt that ideally it *should* be the responsibility of a population to manage its own biology by, for example, wearing protective gloves—but that migrant workers lacked the *suzhi* necessary to be capable of taking on this responsibility (Foucault 1989; Greenhalgh and Winckler 2005; Rose 2006).

Suzhi, according to Yan Hairong (2008), is always expressed as a differential; by asserting that these migrants lacked it, my informants were emphasizing that they in fact had it. Possessing high versus low *suzhi* thus became a hard-and-fast distinction between good and bad migrants. As Jacka (2006) describes, although post-Mao discourses have encouraged the idea that "anyone and everyone can, and should, raise their *suzhi*" (41), for the floating population "this is a status that is even more difficult to change than the Maoist 'bad class' label had been" (42).

The microbes the migrants were thought to carry, meanwhile, became vehicles for the potential transgression of the boundaries between low and high *suzhi* bodies. For many public health professionals, fear of this biological pollution was embodied: Their hands shrank back at the migrants' touch, and they donned protective gear to create barriers between bodies. But no matter what boundaries they were able to erect, the ability of microbial bodies to infect those on both sides of the barrier revealed a shared biological reality that made my interlocutors deeply uncomfortable (Markel 1997; Briggs and Mantini-Briggs 2003).

Professional Boundaries and the Intersubjective Encounter

The structure of China's health system further institutionalized the boundaries drawn between public health professionals and the floating population by limiting the contact that the former had with the latter. Public health institutions and hospitals made up two nonoverlapping *xian* (lines) in the health care system, and public health institutions had little presence in the clinical care environment. Although many of those working in public health complained that these professional boundaries made it difficult to implement some public health interventions, they also told me they were grateful that their own clinical contact was limited, as many had purposefully chosen a field that did not involve dealing directly with sick individuals. Several of my informants had worked in clinical care for years before switching to a career in public health, and they told me that as clinicians they felt burdened by the necessity of "seeing patients" (*kan bingren*). Seeing patients was associated with exhaustion, with frustration, and with their own exploitation. They told me that their clinical physician colleagues were threatened, mistreated, and unappreciated and that by leaving the hospital setting they had escaped a grim existence.

When TM CDC workers occasionally were forced to come into contact with patients or to go to a hospital, they often expressed disgust with the work and with the hospital environment and relief that they did not have to deal with it on a regular basis. On a visit to the main infectious disease hospital that received flu patients during the height of the H1N1 epidemic, for example, Dr. Gong, a forty-year-old TM CDC member who rarely dealt with sick people or with migrants, looked around the ward and declared, "So, this is what it feels like to be a 'real' doctor. Well, I like being a doctor in the office more. There's a funny smell here, it's hot, and so tiring to do this 'real' kind of doctor work; you have to be on your feet all day, and you have to deal with patients, all day patients telling you, 'this hurts,' and 'that hurts'—it's terrible!"

Numerous conversations like this one suggested that many public health professionals not only did not like to interact with migrants, they did not like to interact with sick people at all. In diseased bodies, and in the suffering patients that inhabited them, they saw unpleasant smells, endless complaining, and unwanted responsibilities. Migrant bodies were assumed to be diseased; thus contact with these bodies, even presumably healthy ones, was especially unappealing to my informants.

There is nothing particularly remarkable about this attitude—many people shrink from obligations to engage with the ill or the "backward" in the sort of close physical fashion that is required of physicians, nurses, caregivers, and other clinical professionals. But the rejection of face-to-face contact with individuals that many of my informants exhibited was critical in establishing members of Tianmai's floating population as biological noncitizens, unfit for inclusion in the civilized immigrant common.

Medical anthropologists who study the clinical encounter have shown how moral engagement emerges from the intersubjective encounter between healer and sufferer (Das 2000; Kleinman and Watson 2006), how suffering and healing occurs in the space between two subjects acknowledging each other's humanity (Good 1994; Biehl 2005), and how this recognition of the Other is, in Levinas's words, "the very bond of human subjectivity, even to the point of being raised to a supreme ethical principle" (1988, 159). By avoiding clinical or other personal interactions, public health professionals avoided this intersubjective encounter.[18] And although they avoided this intersubjective encounter with all potential patients—not only members of the the floating population—it was the floating population that was a constant presence in their work and that they therefore had to actively work the hardest to avoid. The kinds of people who made up the common to be served— middle-class, high-*suzhi* people who embodied the image that Tianmai's public health professionals were trying to cultivate for themselves—rarely appeared before them in the flesh as potential patients. Thus the common was able to remain a pristine symbol of the Tianmai dream, untarnished by the messy realities of sweat and blood.

Those who did have contact with migrants in the outpatient clinic were faced with a system that from the start was set up to treat them as a dangerous polluting population. In this encounter, the migrants were not the Other in Levinas's sense of the fellow human but rather the Other in Frantz Fanon's sense of a "nonbeing," stuck in "crushing objecthood" (1986, 109). Much as the medical gaze can reduce an individual in a clinical encounter to his or her pathologies, the gaze of public health professionals in the clinic reduced a line of persons with bodies to a population of biological risk, their bodily processes reinforcing their identities as part of a statistical probability of contagion and failing to render them more human (Foucault 1989; Good 1994).

The volume of people whom public health professionals handled and the assembly-line fashion in which they handled them made it impossible to interact with patients for more than a few seconds at a time. The assumption from the outset was that these few seconds would be aggravating, that the migrant would be incapable of comprehending any but the most simple instructions, and that contact should be minimized in the interest of containing the migrant's inherent contamination. Words other than basic instructions were rarely exchanged, and migrants were chided for asking questions. In this setting it was not really possible for public health professionals to engage seriously with the migrants as human subjects, even if they had wanted to.

It is important to note that critics have for years been identifying a similar problem in the context of the doctor–patient relationship in China (and elsewhere). Physicians in large Chinese cities treat up to 100 patients a day and are accused of carrying out their work "with little regard for their patients' welfare" (Hsiao and Hu 2011, 118). But although in the case of clinical care this behavior was held up as undesirable and unethical by scholars, the media, and ordinary citizens in China, in the case of public health work it was seen as entirely appropriate. Caring for patients is a physician's primary responsibility; as Byron Good (1994) argues, "Caring, exemplified by our idealized vision of medicine, is at the center of our moral discourse. . . . Perhaps this soteriological quality of medicine explains our outrage when physicians fail to live up to these moral standards" (87). But caring is not what public health is supposed to do.

In her discussion of the scientization of global public health interventions, Vincanne Adams (2013) bemoans what she calls the "disappearance of the subject" in public health in favor of dispassionate evaluations of population risk, leading to an "erasure of a critical relationship of caregiving" (85–86). But Tianmai's public health professionals did not see the disappearance of the subject in the populations with which they dealt as a problem because they did not see public health as a caregiving profession. In fact, my interlocutors tended to justify their lack of interest in engaging with individuals by appealing to professional responsibilities. As discussed in the Introduction, Tianmai's public health professionals drew on both Chinese and Western disciplinary divisions to argue that as public health professionals they were charged with protecting the collective, not the individual; the body politic, not individual bodies. As one young woman said, "We do not deal with individuals (*geren*), we deal with crowds (*renqun*), and what we're treating (*zhi*) is population groups (*qunti*). We aren't responsible for treating individuals, that's not what we do." In leaning on existing professional boundaries to concern themselves only with the group, Tianmai's public health profession-als shielded themselves from the suffering of individual migrant lives.

Controlling the Population, Protecting the Common

Sirens scream, and a line of people in white biohazard suits, their faces obscured by hoods and masks, emerge from the back of a van adorned with the green and black logo of the TM CDC. "This is an invisible battlefront," the voiceover drones ominously. More figures in biohazard suits spill out. "When epidemic diseases erupt, they are on the front lines." And then, an idyllic scene of a quiet field of beautifully manicured grass, the kind of well-cared-for green space that is treasured in the *xiaoqu* of the middle class. A smartly dressed elderly couple, pre-sumably grandparents, sit on a swing, a single plump, fresh-faced toddler nestled between them. The characters above and below their heads read, "*shouhu gongmin, jiankang shenghuo*"—"safeguard citizens, have a healthy life." The voiceover re-sumes, "Your health, my commission, is our permanent conviction." The idyllic scene disappears, and foreboding music, as if out of a thriller film, surges. The green and black TM CDC logo swoops victoriously into the center of the screen. The family, it appears, has been saved.

—FROM A PROMOTIONAL VIDEO FOR THE TM CDC

Promotional videos like the one described above presented the TM CDC's public health professionals as heroic virus hunters who would save Tianmai from terrifying threats. The heroics that they exhibited during the malaria epidemics would reappear to once again protect the modern city that they had struggled to build. Though TM CDC workers in the video were shown racing to the scene of an outbreak, however, they were not shown coming into contact with people. Rather, an idealized vision of the *civilized immi-grant common* was seen from afar, its members enjoying the cleanliness and protections that public health professionals had secured for them. The threat to the common, on the other hand, came to be embodied in the invisible presence of the floating population, which jeopardized this scene with its backward germs.

Herein lies the problem with drawing clear professional lines between responsibility for the group and responsibility for the individuals who reside within it. Most members of the floating population, excluded from other sources of health access, rarely interacted with health professionals other than public health clinic workers. These workers, however, embraced personal and political boundaries that excluded the floating population from the group to be served and then embraced professional boundaries that excluded anything but the group level from their concerns.

In establishing a civilized immigrant common as the group to be served, public health professionals established the floating population as the group that could not be served. What made this so insidious was the firmness with which they regarded these boundaries: The floating population was a group who had to repeatedly sacrifice for the good of the common, but who could never reap the benefits. The responsibility of public health professionals vis-à-vis the migrants thus became, more than anything else, a responsibility to keep dangerous intruders under control. In their efforts to fulfill this responsibility, however, my interlocutors remained complicit in the self-defeating principle of biological noncitizenship, which shut migrants out from the very services and care that might have helped them to be healthier, less mobile, and less of a threat to others.

Levinas would argue that in the context of the intersubjective encounter, it is not possible to exclude any single person from one's concerns because "man is responsible for the other man and . . . he is responsible for him even when the other does not concern him, because the other always concerns him" (Raffoul 2010, 203). Mencius, the Confucian sage, argues for a similar type of innate human sense of responsibility to the Other, giving the example of someone observing a child falling down a well: "Now, when men suddenly see a child about to fall into a well, they all have a feeling of alarm and distress; not to gain friendship with the child's parents, nor to seek the praise of their neighbors and friends, nor because they dislike the reputation [of lack of humanity if they did not rescue the child]" (in Tu 1979, 57).

Along these lines, in the case of clinical medicine, Good (1994), Kleinman (1988), Bosk (1981), and others have shown that even when the patient is reduced to his or her pathology, the suffering that the patient is undergoing or may undergo still nags at the clinician who is treating him or her. The healer is still aware of his or her own participation in the moral drama of another's suffering; that healer cannot entirely rid him- or herself of this "soteriological" element. Public health professionals in Tianmai, however, were able to avoid this to a much greater degree by avoiding any intersubjective encounter with the Other. By arguing that intersubjective engagement with patients was not part of their jobs, my informants were able to present their own lack of concern for the well-being of the individuals who came through their clinics as ethical, just, and professionally responsible.

But by building boundaries around their common and then avoiding seeing what Levinas refers to as the "face" of the individuals who overwhelmingly populated Tianmai, my interlocutors in effect avoided having to take responsibility for most of the people living in their city. The result was that Tianmai's public health professionals tended to fulfill neither their professional responsibilities to prevent disease in the "group" nor their personal and moral responsibilities to the Other that Levinas and Mencius would argue they innately had.

Service, Governance, and Self

Historically, the profession of public health has frequently been associated with a call for social justice (Acheson and Fee 1991). One of the most cited definitions of public health in circulation in China when I was doing my fieldwork was one put forth in 1920 by American public health leader Charles-Edward Amory Winslow, who referred to public health as the "Great Crusade" and declared one of the public health profession's primary responsibilities to be "the development of social machinery which will ensure every individual in a community a standard of living adequate for the maintenance of health; so organizing these benefits in such a fashion as to enable every citizen to realize his birthright and longevity" (Acheson and Fee 1991, 5).

Given the high levels of inequality in China's cities and the social justice motivations implied in this and similar definitions of public health, it is worth asking *why* Tianmai's public health professionals did not—in spite of all of the boundaries, fears, and prejudices—commit themselves to serving the floating population. Would not serving this population help to alleviate concerns about instability and disease spread and in turn serve the common as well? Some of my informants agreed that perhaps it would, and they told me that they felt sorry for the floating population and felt sad about the destitute circumstances in which its members lived. But social justice simply was not a motivation for most public health professionals in Tianmai. In fact, many of my interlocutors told me that they had gone into public health expressly to *avoid* having to deal with the types of people who made up the floating population. Having been born into conditions of poverty themselves, they were relieved to have escaped into the middle class. They had no interest in reengaging with the world of poverty and suffering.

The resemblance of the family and green space in the promotional video to my informants' own families and homes was no accident. In saving the middle-class family from the threat of backwardness, Tianmai's public health professionals were also saving one part of their divided selves from the other; in controlling the dangerous population, they were in effect controlling parts of themselves (Kleinman et al. 2011). And so they continued to exclude as they included, reflecting onto the "city of immigrants" only the parts of their divided selves that they wanted to see.

Chapter Two

Relationships, Trust, and Truths

It was two o'clock on a hot Tianmai afternoon in October 2008, and I was drunk, reclining in an easy chair, eating watermelon, and having my feet massaged. I had embarked that morning with several members of the TM CDC parasitology department to conduct a routine inspection of a hospital malaria surveillance system. But what started as a mundane inspection rapidly morphed into a competitive drinking and eating session from which we were all now recovering by having our feet massaged, courtesy of the hospital we had just inspected. After the massage, our hosts treated us to an afternoon "rest" period of *mahjiang* and tea and then to the second banquet of the day, during which everyone made grand declarations of friendship and promised to work together to fight malaria. It wasn't until 9 p.m. that we finally took our leave.

Banqueting and other work-related entertainment events such as these (collectively referred to as *yingchou*) solidified the *guanxi* that public health professionals in Tianmai built with each other. *Guanxi*, often translated as "personal relationships," refers to the reciprocal obligations established between two people in a social network, and social scientists have long considered it to be one of the fundamental organizing principles of Chinese societies (King 1991; Fei 1992; Yang 1994; Yan 1996; Kipnis 1997). As I quickly learned, in Tianmai's public health system nothing—not a vaccination campaign, nor a malaria inspection, nor an AIDS awareness event—happened without *guanxi*.

Aihwa Ong (1999), in her study of globetrotting Chinese elites, found that the Chinese professionals she knew held up *guanxi* as something to be celebrated. *Guanxi* for Ong's informants was a key part of a cohesive collective Chinese identity that lay the basis for the construction of an "alternative modernity" distinct from Western-style Weberian bureaucracy. For the elites who built China's public health system after SARS, however, *guanxi* was an embarrassing and inefficient symbol of traditionalism that necessarily should be replaced.

This chapter is the story of a passionate and laborious attempt on the part of the young, highly educated professionals who streamed into Tianmai's public health institutions after SARS to rid the public health system of a governance process rooted in *guanxi*. In the last chapter we saw how Tianmai's public health professionals sought to govern the floating population in order to protect the *civilized immigrant common* of their Tianmai dream. In this chapter I will show how, in order to more effectively govern the population and thus protect that common, my interlocutors also sought to build and to serve a *professional common*. This common, as they imagined it, would mirror what they thought they knew about how Western professionals related to each other. The professional common would be led by an educated scientific elite, would be guided by rationality and truth, and would be rooted in what I call *professionalized trust*—a form of bounded social trust shared among colleagues that the new public health professionals hoped would supplant personalistic trust built through *guanxi*.

Only a *guanxi*-free professional common, Tianmai's public health reformers told me, could produce the kind of effective governance needed to protect their city, their country, and the world from twenty-first-century population health threats. Serving a professional common thus ultimately meant serving many other commons. But serving a professional common also was an end in itself. After SARS those who worked in public health sought to establish public health in China as a globally relevant, scientific profession. Committing themselves to their vision of the professional common, they imagined, was the first step in achieving this goal.

As with all iterations of the common, the object of service here was an idealized *group* rather than an individual. Public health projects previously had been implemented only via the personal networks that individual public health workers built with each other. It was only after carefully nurturing a *guanxi* relationship with a key collaborator or collaborators that one might attempt to implement a vaccination campaign or HIV intervention. The dyadic nature of the relationship was critical: In agreeing at the end of a shared meal to assist in implementing a program, a *guanxi* partner signaled a commitment to serve the specific other person involved in this activity.

In establishing a professional common, however, Tianmai's public health professionals hoped that all those working in and for public health would implement projects on behalf of an abstract collegial group. To do this, everyone had to be prepared to take instructions from anonymous colleagues with whom they did not necessarily have a relationship. They also were expected to produce results that corresponded not to what a particular *guanxi* partner wanted but rather to what the professional common needed. And first and foremost what the professional common needed, the new public health professionals insisted, were two things: accurate biostatistics that provided scientific truths about the population and a reliable means of sharing those statistics. Effective control of diseases in the population would, they thought, naturally emerge from the accomplishment of these two goals.

The new public health professionals expected both their colleagues and themselves to accomplish all of these goals without raising a single glass. Professional ideals, rather than the rules of *guanxi*, were to motivate people to do their work. The erasure of *guanxi* relationships, however, proved to be both exceedingly difficult to accomplish and dubiously effective in producing results.

One of the factors that made erasing *guanxi* so difficult was the tension inside the TM CDC between those who sought to abolish *guanxi* and those who insisted on its value. This was more than a procedural distinction—it was a matter of great ethical import. For *guanxi* defenders, *guanxi* relationships were not just expedient tools of governance. They also were the only means through which many of the older members of the public health world felt they could trust others or ethically serve them. The reciprocal commitments formed through *guanxi* partnerships grew out of the Confucian ethical principle of *renqing*, or "human feelings," and produced what Ellen Oxfeld (2010) calls *liangxin*—the remembering and acting upon of moral obligations.

The new public health professionals attempted to replace personalistic ethics based in *renqing* and *liangxin* with a more abstract ethic of generalized responsibility based in professionalized trust. Service to the professional common should be motivated by a commitment to science and a sense of responsibility to the production of "truth," they told me. It should be demonstrated through the production of data that met biomedical, rather than *guanxi*-based, standards of truth. Science was to render relationships, and their ethics, irrelevant. When it failed to do so, Tianmai's public health professionals found themselves lodged uncomfortably between the fantasy of the professional common and the necessity of the banquet hall.

Guanxi *and Governance*

General standards have no utility. The first thing to do is to understand the specific context: Who is the important figure, and what kind of relationship is appropriate with that figure? Only then can one decide the ethical standards to be applied in that context.

—FEI XIAOTONG (1992, 78)

To understand why *guanxi* was so important and so difficult to replace, we first need to understand the critical role it played in allowing public health professionals to govern their populations. Public health projects at the local level in China often began with a symbolic gesture from a central government leader. Dr. Tang, who ran outreach programs for the TM CDC's HIV/AIDS department, for example, told me that one such symbolic gesture made shortly after the SARS epidemic was the reason that HIV/AIDS became the focus of an entire department at the TM CDC. "[Premier] Wen Jiabao went and shook hands with AIDS patients. He didn't shake hands with hepatitis patients," he told me. "So when a leader that high up does that, the lower levels have no choice—they have to start prioritizing whatever the higher leader signals they should prioritize."[1]

Making sure that the leader's will was done was not a simple exercise in authoritarian power, however. Due to China's system of "fragmented authoritarianism" (Lieberthal 1995), the central government had little practical ability to force local level governments to implement its policies, whereas local governments often had little ability to compel their associated institutions to work together (Zhong 2003). Local public health institutions, meanwhile, lacked jurisdiction, legal or otherwise, over those on whom they depended to carry out projects (Zhang et al. 2012). "The biggest problem with the system is that we have no power [*quanli*] to make the lower levels listen," Dr. Du, a microbiologist involved with many cooperative projects, told me.

The power to implement a project instead lay within the overlapping *guanxi* webs that the relevant people, institutions, and ideas conjured. Each time a program was implemented, the webs reentangled in novel ways. It was these entanglements themselves that made things happen, convinced people that they should happen, and provided the moral framework that guided what happened and how. *Guanxi* relationships thus were the only means by which my informants could enact any of the dozens of public health directives issued by the local BOH each month, as well as any projects of their own conceiving. These relationships also shaped hierarchies within each work unit, or *danwei*: Those who banqueted well, and built good *guanxi*, were promoted more frequently and rapidly than those who did not.

Public health professionals in Tianmai, Guangzhou, and elsewhere thus frequently told me that the most critical parts of their jobs took place after hours in social settings. Dr. Gong told me in an interview: "Those of us working at these government institutions always have two jobs that we have to juggle: One is to complete our tasks (*yewu*) and the other is to build *guanxi* . . . to get the support (*zhichi*) to do the tasks." That is why, she said, they had to spend more time with "friends" (*pengyou*) than with family (*jiaren*). "We rarely go home after work and spend time with family; we always have to go out with friends, because we need the friends," she told me.

As Gong implied, nurturing enough *guanxi* in enough of the right places could be a time-consuming and complex process. As in other big cities, the Tianmai City CDC presided over a larger local CDC system that included institutions at the "district" (*qu*), "street" (*jiedao*), and "community" (*shequ*) levels. The system had a "*kuai-kuai*" (horizontal) structure (Lieberthal 1995; Zhong 2003), in that at each level the CDC was under the jurisdiction of the corresponding BOH, which exercised control over all hires, projects, and campaigns and provided funding. At the same time, it had a "*tiao-tiao*" (vertical) structure of "technical direction" that was supposed to flow from city CDC to district CDCs to street-level CDCs, community health service

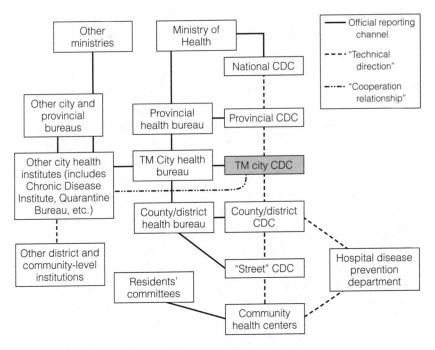

Figure 2.1. Tianmai's public health system (as of 2009).
Created by the author.

centers, and hospital disease control departments or *fangbao ke* (these were located in hospitals but were part of the public health rather than clinical system).[2,3] As one informant put it, "*tiao shi guan yewu, kuai shi guan qian* [*tiao* handles the work, *kuai* handles the money]." (See Figure 2.1.)

The TM CDC also received technical direction from CDCs at the provincial and central levels, though because of the TM CDC's strong technical and financial capacities, it often felt free to ignore it. This made *guanxi* all the more important if national and provincial CDCs wanted to work with Tianmai. The relative independence of even district- and street-level CDCs in the city meant that the city TM CDC was equally dependent on *guanxi* to gain the cooperation of the lower levels.

Because the CDC was one of perhaps a dozen city institutions with some public health–related functions—some of them under the jurisdiction of the BOH, some under other city bureaus, and some under central or provincial control—it also had "cooperation" (*hezuo*) relationships with these other institutions on a project-by-project basis. In addition, many of the functions of the CDC were redundant with other government *danweis*. For example, at the time of my fieldwork food safety was managed by five different city bureaus and institutes, each of which focused on one aspect of the food production cycle. All of this made for a somewhat chaotic public health governance structure.

When a public health directive arrived at a local CDC in the form of a *wenjian* (official document), the first step was to decide whether it was "crucial" (Zhong 2003) and thus worthy of investing time and resources. My informants told me that they made this determination based partially on how much the leaders one level above were pushing the project, partially on how much the project might benefit the *danwei*, partially on how much face (*mianzi*) CDC leaders were likely to lose by *not* implementing the directive or to gain by implementing it well, and partially on whether the project was likely to be successful. Directives that did not pass the initial relevance test were not considered to be worth the effort of *guanxi* building: This was the difference, as was explained to me, between *kai hui* (holding a meeting) and *zuo shi* (doing things). The least important directives were passed down to the lower levels as another *wenjian*. If a directive seemed slightly more important, a meeting might be held to state the necessity of carrying out the project. Neither of these actions on its own was likely to elicit much response.

When a directive was determined to be crucial, however, more action needed to be taken. This was where *guanxi* not only could but *must* come in if the project was to have any chance of being implemented. BOH leaders had to use their *guanxi* with parallel CDC leaders to entrust the latter group with the project; the CDC leaders in turn relied on whatever webs of *guanxi* connections were at their disposal to implement it. When done well, this created the appearance of a tight hierarchical system with clear lines of power that could efficiently enforce policy from top to bottom.

Consider the case of measles control. In 2005, WHO's Western Pacific Region established a target date of 2012 for the elimination of measles from the region, which includes China. This goal was to be accomplished primarily through increased vaccination coverage. WHO named China as the country carrying the highest disease burden in the region, and the central government made lowering the measles infection rate a top priority. "When WHO gives the final report in 2012, China cannot still have a high measles rate," one woman explained to me. "The leaders will lose a lot of face if we can't show that we made more progress than anyone else in the region. So there is a lot of pressure on us to make sure this happens."[4]

In response, in 2008, the Guangdong provincial BOH issued a directive announcing a campaign for the "strengthening of measles vaccine immunization," and the TM BOH followed with a similar notice in early 2009. For one month in the spring of 2009, the TM CDC was to mobilize lower-level institutions to ensure that every child in Tianmai between the ages of eight months and fourteen years received a measles vaccine, regardless of his or her vaccination history or Tianmai residency status. This was a compelling directive to implement because of post-SARS promises to protect a global common from China's infectious diseases. "We are supposed to fight it like we fought SARS," one of the women running the campaign at the TM CDC told me in an interview.

The urgency with which the leaders approached the measles campaign, however, had only tenuous connections to the disease burden in Tianmai. Although measles was a more serious problem in Tianmai than in other large cities in Guangdong, through prevention and vaccination programs already in place the TM CDC reported that the number of measles cases in Tianmai in 2008 had already fallen 60 percent from 2007 levels and was now at a level of twenty-six cases per 100,000 population—well below the figures for hepatitis or tuberculosis, neither of which got its own campaign. Furthermore, though the mobility of the floating population meant that frequent vaccination campaigns were necessary to cover all of the children who cycled in and out of the city, a 100 percent vaccination policy would result in thousands of children being unnecessarily revaccinated—many of them after having just been vaccinated as part of the previous year's campaign. Thus in their determination to reach the WHO target, Tianmai's public health professionals embarked on a redundant campaign against a disease that by their own account was already in retreat in Tianmai. That did not bother most TM CDC members working on the campaign: Using resources efficiently was not on the top of their list of priorities.

I accompanied members of the TM CDC vaccination department as they mobilized their *guanxi* networks to implement this directive. The first thing they did was to visit each of the six district CDCs in Tianmai with an entourage that included the department head or vice department head, a driver, and several department members or students. A personal visit from someone of importance from the city-level CDC signaled to the district leaders that this was something that the city leaders prioritized. As several informants explained to me, the closer to one's level (district, street) a leader is, the more likely one is to take notice of what he or she is advocating. Thus, while the district CDC might not pay much attention to whether the provincial leaders were prioritizing measles, if the city CDC leader declared its importance, the district listened.

After a polite meeting in which everyone declared their mutual appreciation for the hard work of the others, the district leader took us to see some of his friends at two street-level CDCs. The leaders of the street CDCs in turn accompanied the whole group to the institutions that would be charged with actually administering the vaccinations, including community health service centers, vaccination stations, *juweihui* (residents' committees), community (*shequ*) committees, and *liudong renkou chuzuwu guanli suo* (floating population rental management bureaus) to seek their support.[5]

Two aspects of this process are particularly important to note. First, *guanxi* networks expanded outward via a chain of dyadic relationships (Fei 1992). That is, at the center of each network was a face-to-face relationship between two individuals. Any collective effects that emerged had to be grounded in these collections of interpersonal exchanges. Second, at every level, the *guanxi* connections for a given person were mostly limited to a select group one level lower than the initiator of the interaction. Thus, the city-level CDC workers had connections with certain people at each of the district CDCs, but they rarely had direct *guanxi* connections with those at the community or street level. The district CDC workers had connections with workers at *some* of the street CDCs but rarely with the community level. And usually only those at the residents' committees and community health service centers directly interacted with local populations. Thus not only did the city-level CDC workers rely entirely on the district CDCs' *guanxi* webs, and the district CDCs in turn relied on the *guanxi* of the street level and so on, but those webs were limited and constantly in flux depending on which particular people were called on one level below. The key point here is that the whole system turned on dyadic interactions between specific individuals who had personal relationships with each other. Hierarchy played a role, but only in the sense that a high-up leader normally had many friends. His power was derived from those friendships and was entirely dependent on them.

On our initial district visit, for example, the district CDC leader took us to a street-level department run by what he described as one of his closest friends. This friend then took us to see a friend at one of the nearby residents' committees. Everyone then retired for an early lunch attended by members of the street, district, and city CDCs, which involved toasting and drinking to confirm everyone's cooperation in the deal. We then were all invited for a foot massage at the expense of the street-level department before making the long trip back to the city CDC. Satisfied that enough members of that district were on board, the next day we went to another district and repeated the same exercise. Several months later, my contact in the vaccination department told me that she had reported 100 percent compliance in the vaccination campaign.

If these numbers seem too good to be true, this is because they often were. From the standpoint of *guanxi*-based expectations, the willingness to satisfy the obligations inherent to a personal relationship between "friends" was more important than producing numbers that were "true" (Kuhn 1962; Shapin 1994; Blum 2007). Most people I knew assumed that the numbers that the lower levels produced rarely represented the actual number of vaccines administered. From the standpoint of *guanxi*-based relationships, this was not very important: As Susan Blum (2007) has argued, the production of data was itself seen "as a sincere attempt to please and meet the expectations of the receiver" and thus producing data that met these expectations was more important than producing data that corresponded to what the *guanxi* partner "really" did (68). The expectation in this case was that the vaccination campaign would be successful, and so success was what was reported. "Truth" in the sense of simple correspondence, whereby knowledge produced about the world was supposed to map perfectly onto the facts "as they really are" (Kuhn 1962) was different from being true to one's *guanxi* partner.

The discordance between these two versions of truth produced tensions between those who celebrated *guanxi* and those who maligned it. For the latter group, the failure of *guanxi*-produced truth to be "scientific" was deceptive and unethical. But for the former group, to produce a scientific truth that violated the expectations of a *guanxi* relationship would be a brazen breach of an important ethical ritual.

Rituals of Guanxi

The definition of public health in China is networking, that is, you have to use their language to talk, and that language is to get drunk. . . . In China if you want to do anything, you need to talk first. There are a lot of opportunities for talking, but timing is everything; you have to wait for the opportune moment. And that opportune moment is usually when you're drunk, falling down drunk, or tipsy, or at least blurry, or even losing consciousness, at least when your consciousness is not so good, at these times the distance between people is very close. And then when you tell him something, he'll think, this is my friend, and he'll remember.

—XU DAN, EPIDEMIOLOGIST AT TM CDC

The rituals that shaped *guanxi* interactions in the public health setting—primarily in the form of banquets—were seen as not only *logistically* necessary but also *ethically* necessary for any project to proceed. The rituals produced, and were guided by, a type of intersubjective work called *renqing*, or "human feelings" (Yang 1994; Yan 1996). As Yan (1996) describes in the case of villagers in northeastern China, the *renqing* ethics that accompany *guanxi* relationships serve "as an important standard by which villagers judge whether one is a proper social person" (225). Kleinman (1995) describes *renqing* as "both social and deeply personal; it captures the dialectical quality of experience; it is individual and interpersonal. It represents the moral core of experience" (111). Someone who recognizes and nurtures *renqing* between him- or herself and another person effectively accepts responsibility toward that individual. This in turn produces a form of what Ellen Oxfeld (2010) calls *liangxin*, or "conscience." According to Oxfeld, having *liangxin* means remembering what others have done and then acting on that obligation by returning a favor in the future. Although Oxfeld does not see *guanxi* as a prerequisite for *liangxin*, *guanxi* rituals nurtured the *liangxin*-like obligations that made Tianmai's public health system function.

Kwang-kuo Hwang (1987) points out that most *guanxi* connections involve a mix of instrumental and affective ties, but it is the affective ties that bind people together. Instrumentality without affection veers close to corruption and removes the meaning from the interaction and the longevity from the tie (Yan 1996). Despite my informants' often instrumental goals, those who excelled at banqueting told me that they relied heavily on the affective side of *guanxi*. Without human feelings, they said, how would they know that those in other work units or departments would help them—and that they would help again in the future?

The production of *renqing* was dependent on the correct enactment of *"li"* (etiquette, or ritual). From a Confucian point of view, principles of *li* guided all aspects of human relatedness, from basic everyday interactions to sacred reciprocal responsibilities including filial piety, as well as *guanxi* relationships (Tu 1979, 1985; Yang 1994). According to neo-Confucian scholar Tu Wei-ming (1979), the cultivation of *ren* (humaneness, benevolence) in turn guided *li*: "*Li* becomes empty formalism if *ren* is absent. Furthermore, *li* without *ren* easily degenerates into social coercion incapable of conscious improvement and liable to destroy any true human feelings" (13).

My informants told me that principles of *li* underlay the structure of the banquets and the rules of the gift giving that drove their *guanxi* interactions—including who sat where in a banquet, who toasted first, and who incurred which obligations to whom. Attempting to implement a project without going through proper *guanxi* channels or performing proper rituals meant transgressing *li*. This was both unethical and terribly ineffective. Such attempts would normally be ignored, rebuffed, or at best performed halfheartedly. If the rituals were performed correctly, on the other hand, they would in theory create *renqing* in the space between the people involved in the ritual and with that an ethical responsibility to help each other.

Banquets constituted the primary rituals through which Tianmai's public health professionals built and maintained *guanxi*. In a typical banquet, the host opened by leading a toast to everyone at the table, before toasting the guest of honor (such as a visiting leader) and emptying his or her glass. Then the rest of the people at the table toasted the guest. Once the guest of honor had been toasted, each person at the table had to toast each other person individually, usually starting with the host and other leaders, and working his or her way to less important guests or colleagues. Once a participant toasted someone, that person was obligated to return the toast. If there was more than one table, the leaders got up and toasted all the other tables, and these people later reciprocated in groups. By an hour into any serious banquet, the entire banquet hall will have broken down into an endless cycle of toasting, with all guests on their feet circulating to make sure they toasted everyone the correct number of times. Once the host was satisfied that the guests had been duly celebrated and that enough *renqing* had been established to assure cooperation, then the host issued one final toast to the table or room and closed the banquet. Rarely would this happen before everyone was thoroughly intoxicated (see Mason 2013).

The rules governing who paid for a banquet and the lavishness of the food, setting, and alcohol were quite involved. According to one interlocutor who participated in banquets at least twice a week, "The lower levels always treat the upper levels, but they only do a really *reqing* [enthusiastic] job if the *guanxi* is really good. . . . If the *guanxi* is good, the standard is about 150 RMB/person, but for a more important leader, it's 300 RMB/person . . . But if your *guanxi* is bad, maybe only 30 RMB/person." *Guanxi* thus builds on itself—if the *guanxi* is good, then a more lavish banquet follows, and more opportunities emerge for building even better *guanxi*.

The interesting thing about the economics of banqueting in the public health setting is that the same party seeking to benefit was more often than not the one being treated to the banquet as well. Thus higher-level CDCs usually visited lower levels to convince the lower levels to cooperate on a project, but it was actually the lower-level CDCs that then usually treated the higher levels to a banquet. The higher levels reciprocated by giving the lower levels face—agreeing to attend the banquet, bringing enough of an entourage, giving the lower-level leader the seat of honor, and ensuring that everyone properly toasted the leader and his subordinates.[6] But it was *ren-qing*, born of the alcohol-laden revelry, that secured the relationship and bound the two sides to each other. The lower level would help the upper level because its members were now ethically bound to each other as friends.

In most instances, the sharing of food and drink at a banquet was key to the building of *renqing*. One felt one's obligations to the other with the whole of oneself, via a shared embodied memory (Kipnis 2002). Judith Farquhar (2002) describes her experience of embodiment in this way:

> By the end of the evening, I had drunk more liquor than ever before. I felt quite lucid, though not entirely in command of all my limbs, and I loved these men . . . we were linked by something more substantive, a pleasantly shared moment in our lives. This comradeship [*ganqing*] existed . . . as a foundation for continued negotiations that would match our respective offerings and requirements (excesses and deficiencies) in working relationships." (151)

For Farquhar, the visceral effects of alcohol were critical for creating bonds through the banqueting ritual. "One must actually raise one's glass to show respect for one's companions, and one must actually drink the liquor to find carnal, emotional, and spiritual commonality with them," Farquhar writes (2000, 151–152; see also Kipnis 2002). Avid banqueters whom I knew agreed that the sensation of imbibing alcohol and feeling its effects was essential to benefiting from a banquet. "The culture of alcohol (*jiu wenhua*) is very important in China," a middle-aged leader of a street-level CDC lectured to me at one banquet. "When we drink alcohol, our body feels very comfortable (*shufu*) and then we feel very close to each other (*shuxi*)." The shared phenomenological experience of getting drunk together linked the creation of friendship and its benefits with a loss of mental and bodily control (Csordas 1993; Mason 2013). Sentiment was formed through altered consciousness, and feelings of connectedness grew as a result.[7]

For many of my younger interlocutors, however, this elaborate embodied ritual was a waste of time. When they participated in banquets these public health professionals did develop a sense of obligation to help *guanxi* partners—but they insisted that this could easily be accomplished in other ways. As one exasperated epidemiologist told me, "I wish we could just send a fax instead." Establishing a less personal, more professional relationship was seen as more efficient and more dignified. But the focus that the post-SARS newcomers had on efficiency was a bewildering goal for many of the TM CDC's older workers, who had long seen the expenditure of time on *guanxi* rituals as a currency to be maximized rather than minimized. For them, the profoundly embodied experience of serving their "friends" made service to an abstract professional common difficult to even envision.

Guanxi *and* Chuangshou

Some of the staunchest defenders of *guanxi* rituals were those who had for decades been conducting sanitation inspections in Tianmai's restaurants, hotels, and saunas. As the central and local governments retreated from funding public health in the early 1980s, they passed laws allowing public health institutions to fund themselves. In Tianmai, the AES and later the CDC had the legal right to compel all "service" businesses—including restaurants, hotels, saunas, and movie theaters—to pay up to several thousand yuan several times a year for inspections of their kitchenware, towels, air-conditioning vents, swimming pools, and ambient air quality.[8] In addition, all service industry workers were required to carry a health certificate attesting that they were free of infectious diseases. This certificate was provided only on passing a paid physical exam at an approved local clinic; local CDCs hosted many of these clinics (see Chapter One). The TM CDC also made money by selling vaccines and disinfection materials.

By the time SARS arrived, these money-making activities, collectively referred to as *chuangshou*, had become quite lucrative, contributing to a marked rise in *danwei* salaries. *Chuangshou* profits were distributed across the TM CDC, but high-earning departments and team leaders were also amply rewarded, providing incentives for each team to cover as many businesses per day as possible.

I spent approximately one month during the course of my fieldwork working with sanitation inspectors, who made up the bulk of the TM CDC's *chuangshou* staff, trying to understand their roles in the new world of public health in Tianmai. As expected, this involved a good deal of banqueting. The first time I went on a sanitation inspection with Dr. Wu, an inspector in his fifties with twenty-five years of experience, I committed a terrible faux pas. It was nearing noon, and we were on our way to a high-end dim sum restaurant that would be our next stop. Wu suggested cheerfully that I must be learning a lot about China from my experience doing inspections, and I said, equally cheerfully, "Yes, and also eating a lot of good free food!" There was silence in the car, and the other team members looked out the window. Wu turned around from the front passenger seat and looked at me, hard. "No, the food is not free," he told me. "These are friends who *qing ke* [treat us to lunch] because we are all *shou* [close]."

As a restaurant inspector who excelled at *chuangshou*, Dr. Wu had the chance to make a lot of friends. The daily routine for the restaurant inspection team usually included a morning visit to one or two mess halls, followed by a noodle house or other inexpensive eatery, and then a noontime arrival at a five-star restaurant. The team leader—generally an older man with many years of experience—would ask for one of the managers by name (who would have been warned that morning that we were coming), and we would be whisked off to a private room. The manager and our leader would greet each other like old friends. We would ask to see the kitchenware that we were to be swabbing for bacteria, a request that was almost always met with the protest, "First rest awhile, and have a little lunch!" Our team leader would agree that we could not very well do the inspection hungry. This usually would be followed by a lavish meal, which sometimes escalated into a raucous drinking session. After we had eaten and drunk our fill, sparkling sets of dishes would be brought out for inspection. (See Figure 2.2.)

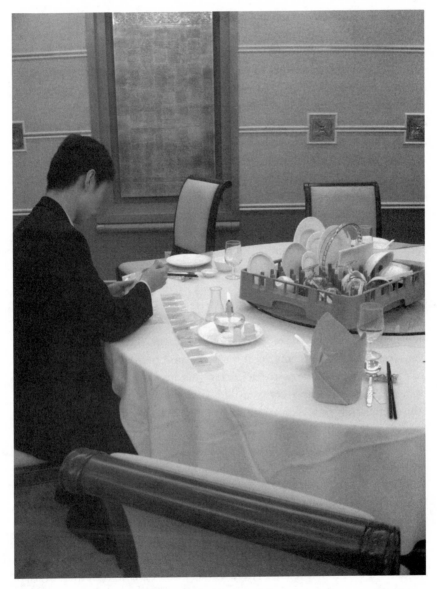

Figure 2.2. Sanitation inspection at a restaurant in Tianmai, 2009.
Photo by the author.

The inspectors whom I accompanied told me that it was important to build good *guanxi* with the high-end restaurant owners, because the TM CDC was asking them to pay a lot of money for several inspections a year, many of which were redundant with those conducted by other institutions. As in the case of the banqueting performed with other public health *danweis*, good *guanxi* established a set of reciprocal obligations. The restaurant owners helped the inspectors by serving food and helping to fill a quota and produce income for the TM CDC. The inspectors in turn would accept whatever highly sanitized items were brought to them. They would warn that they were coming and would serve as allies should they be called in to do a food poisoning investigation in the future.[9] As in Oxfeld's descriptions of *liangxin*, memory was important here. The inspectors would remember the delicious meals they were served, and the restaurant owners would remember the lenience they were granted—thus committing both parties to a long-term mutual obligation to protect and serve. Despite appearances, however, in the eyes of Dr. Wu and his colleagues none of these acts constituted bribery— because all of them were compelled by *renqing* ethics established between two people experiencing the pleasures of eating and drinking together.[10]

The more lunches I attended, the more I realized what Wu meant when he said that the lunches were a case of "friends treating friends." The manager and Wu did seem close that day: She poured us tea, and he inquired after her business; they talked about housing prices, common acquaintances, plans for the upcoming holiday. It was the expert performance of *guanxi* rituals that assured all those participating that lunch among friends was not bribery. Remembering and rewarding kindness from a friend was not an ethical violation—it was an ethical requirement. This was the source of Wu's discomfort with my calling the food we ate "free." Free food is anonymous, an instrumental attempt to bribe an official. Being treated to lunch is personal, an invitation issued out of affection. Wu always asked for certain managers by name and would accept food only from those with whom he already had a relationship. The difference between the anonymous and the personal became the difference between corruption and friendship.

Although the inspection lunches were usually more casual than the banquets described in the previous section, the form of these interactions—and the declarations of friendship—were similar. The goals were similar as well: to meet the expectations of a *guanxi* partner. It did not much matter whether the plates and cups were actually clean because carrying out the inspection was a goal in itself, and the *guanxi* rituals accomplished this goal quite successfully. The local people who were supposed to benefit from making sure the dishes were free from bacteria did not figure into this, unless they became embodied in the form of a friend going to a restaurant that the inspectors deemed unclean. (I would always be warned against going to certain restaurants, because I was a "friend.")

The distinction between *guanxi* and bribery is one that is common to many societies, especially postsocialist ones. According to Joseph Berliner, the difference between bribery and *blat*, a Soviet practice similar to *guanxi*, is that with *blat* "there is a 'personal basis for expecting a proposal to be listened to,' whereas bribery is conceived of as only a relationship linked by material interest and characterized by direct and immediate payment" (quoted in Yang 1994, 202). Yan (1996) similarly points out that the gifts and other acts exchanged through *guanxi* interactions serve "to sustain a long-term order of social life rather than a short-term personal benefit" (226). It is also the concrete, face-to-face sociality that sets *guanxi* apart from bribery. The fact that Dr. Wu interacted with Ms. Hu, and not Mr. He or Ms. Wang, was key to a successful *guanxi* interaction. The same thing could not be accomplished if any part of the interaction was generalized or disembodied from the specific individuals involved.

The new public health professionals who came to Tianmai after SARS, however, argued that *guanxi* no longer could be distinguished from corruption. Having rejected the primary importance of *renqing*, they effectively rejected this distinction. *Guanxi* interactions became what they looked like on the surface: instrumental transactions that bought influence or power.

Guanxi in service of *chuangshou* was particularly maligned. After SARS, an inverse correlation began to emerge between the prestige of a department and the proportion of the department's personnel who were dedicated to *chuangshou*. SARS hammered home the idea that "we are not here to raise money, we are here to control disease," several informants explained. One young epidemiologist who worked on infectious disease surveillance told me, "Before, we counted on the inspections and the physicals in the clinics, and from my perspective this was nonsense, this kind of work. We should be doing surveillance, reports, working on the management level . . . This is the kind of thing that U.S. CDC does. This doesn't involve *chuangshou*. *Chuangshou* is really the lowest level."[11] Not only were the older workers wasting the CDC's time on unnecessary sanitation inspections, my younger informants told me, they were also prioritizing *guanxi* relationships over building a safe and civilized Tianmai.

These misplaced priorities, they implied, impeded the building of what Yan Yunxiang (2009) calls social trust (see the Introduction). Dr. Wu and Ms. Hu could rely on each other to fulfill their reciprocal obligations, but neither considered their obligations to the strangers who ate at Ms. Hu's restaurant. This fact was not lost on Tianmai's restaurant goers: Friends of mine outside the public health world already assumed that even expensive restaurants might not be clean, due precisely to the problem of *guanxi*. They thus preferred to eat at restaurants where they already knew and trusted people themselves.

In maligning *guanxi* and condemning *chuangshou*, highly educated public health professionals in their twenties and thirties carefully distinguished themselves from older, less educated sanitation inspectors like Dr. Wu who were "too fond of *yingchou*" (*tai xihuan yingchou*). My young informants told me that as professional people (*zhuanye renyuan*) who "had an education" (*duguo shu*), they could and should be trusted to do away with the corrupt practices of the past.

Bring in the New

It was a miserably hot July morning, and I sat sweating in a spacious but humid office at the newly renovated Di'yi District CDC in Tianmai, my legs sticking to a voluminous rolling leather chair. As I talked with Dr. Guo, who headed both the public hygiene and infectious disease departments here, I sipped a delicious brew of high-end *tieguanyin* tea and admired the half dozen bouquets of pink roses wrapped in brightly colored crepe paper that almost entirely covered the surface of Guo's desk. "It is my birthday," Guo explained, skipping around the office, pointing out the view and the mahogany furniture, as she set up a tea set on the elegant coffee table and poured hot water between the slats of the tray. "Everyone knows I love roses. Isn't that thoughtful?"

I was interviewing Guo about her work fighting the H1N1 influenza outbreak, a project of which she was very proud (see Chapter Four). She said that all of the *zhuanye renyuan* (professionals/experts) at her *danwei*—of whom she said there were exactly forty-seven—participated in an emergency management training a few months earlier, just in time for this event. I asked her who counted as *zhuanye*. "Those who *duguo shu* [have some education]," she said. She shook her head, leaning over to pour more hot water into and over the small ceramic teapot, and then refilling my tiny cup. It's a shame, one-third of people in the Di'yi CDC haven't *duguo shu*, she told me.

Guo told me that when her *danwei* first formed in the early 1980s, it was willing to take anyone: no requirements, no standards. So the *danwei* filled with people who had no education, and twenty-five years later those people were still here, waiting to retire. Only five out of twelve of the people in her department were *zhuanye renyuan*. "The rest are just manual laborers; all they know how to do is the same rote testing; you give them something else to do, and they don't understand. They have a lot of experience doing that one thing, but you can't expect them to analyze anything or do any *real* projects," she told me. It was only later that Guo admitted that she had started her career with only a *zhongzhuan* [vocational high school] degree herself, before going back to school in her thirties to complete a bachelor's degree.[12]

Heeding the call of Vice Premier Wu Yi to "train high-*suzhi* [quality] public health management and technical talent" in the wake of SARS, Tianmai's leaders sought to rapidly rectify what Guo found to be wrong with the quality of CDC personnel. City-, district-, and street-level CDCs hired dozens of young people in their twenties and thirties who not only had *"duguo shu"* but who had postgraduate degrees in subjects like epidemiology and molecular biology that were associated with modern scientific public health approaches.

Educational requirements for new members applying to enter the city-level CDC in Tianmai rose from a technical degree (*dazhuan* or *zhongzhuan*) before SARS to a bachelor's degree immediately after. In 2006, the BOH appointed Director Lan as head of the TM CDC; on his arrival Lan further increased the educational requirements for entrance to the CDC to a master's degree and aggressively recruited PhD students and graduates. Ranks within the *danwei* began to be tied to the level of the National Health Professional Skills Qualification Exam (*quanguo weisheng zhuanye jishu zige kaoshi*) that employees had passed.[13] Lan himself had a PhD from one of China's best medical colleges, and two new vice directors, as well as the Party Secretary, all had master's degrees. Some predicted that a PhD would eventually be required just to enter the TM CDC. Members who lacked these higher degrees scrambled to get into part-time master's programs or to at least complete bachelor's degrees, concerned they would be removed from their posts and replaced with someone with less experience but more education—a fate that befell many. A premium also was put on education abroad. The TM CDC's move toward meritocracy especially benefited women, several of whom told me they had been admitted to the *danwei* based on high exam scores alone, without the *guanxi* procedures that many of their older male counterparts had used to secure a similar spot (see Mason 2013).

Thanks to the large amount of local and international funding that the TM CDC enjoyed after SARS, Lan was able to do this hiring at a pace that exceeded most other cities. He was helped by a 370 million RMB grant from the local Tianmai government made in the wake of SARS to build a massive and sparkling new facility in the foothills at the edge of the city that nearly doubled the size of the TM CDC's laboratory and office space and housed top-of-the-line laboratory equipment—all of which made the *danwei* more competitive in attracting scientific talent (Zhang et al. 2008). The institution moved to the new facility in late 2010.

Many of Lan's new recruits were disappointed, however, when on arrival at the TM CDC they found that *guanxi*-building activities like banqueting were nonetheless required to perform their jobs and that a failure to banquet well made job advancement difficult. Lisa Hoffman, in her 2010 study of young urban professionals in China, argues that students graduating from universities in the late reform period assumed that they would automatically benefit from the social mobility that they felt their education owed to them—and that such mobility would follow "rational" and meritocratic processes. This is not entirely what happened at public health institutions in Tianmai. Xiao Chen, a young woman who arrived at the TM CDC shortly after completing her bachelor's degree, told me one afternoon after an exhausting *guanxi*-building lunch, "When I first got here I [already] had to banquet sometimes, and I hated it—I told my father, I didn't study in university for five years so that I could go drinking! There's a saying that to be an official, you need the 'three cans': 'can speak, can write, can drink.'" Even though she excelled at the first two "cans," a failure to excel at the last still held back her advancement, Xiao Chen told me. It was this seeming injustice that drove a lot of the anti-*guanxi* backlash among the young, high-*suzhi* professionals recruited after SARS.[14]

The Professional and the Technician

The dispute over the value of banqueting and *guanxi*, the rapid promotion of well-educated but inexperienced young people to the top of the hierarchy and the devaluing of sanitation work combined to strain relations among *danwei* members. My younger informants often did not disguise their low regard for some of the more poorly educated members of the *danwei* or their feelings that "the professional is the natural ruler of the professional-technical team" (Kultgen 1988, 80–81). The distinction between professional and technician (*jishu renyuan*) became critical: Technicians who ran bacteria samples in the lab, conducted inspections, and completed paperwork were not scientists and were not always treated with respect by those who were (see Shapin 1994). During several of my rotations I went out on project assignments with teams led by recent bachelor's or master's graduates who were in charge of middle-aged members who had previously run the team for years. The older people, having suffered a loss of face at this reversal of traditional hierarchies, seemed unhappy but unwilling to complain (Ikels 2004). Instead they made repeated comments to me about how *"congming"* (clever) their new bosses were and how I should interview these clever people instead of themselves because, as Dr. Wu put it, "They are the ones who are impressive." Their younger superiors, anxious to prove themselves, in turn were often bossy toward older team members, as well as toward support staff with whom these older members had labored to build *guanxi* over many years.

Dr. Qu and Dr. Rong epitomized this new tension. Qu, who was in his late twenties, had a master's degree in environmental science and had taken several PhD courses at a British university—an experience that he repeatedly recounted to anyone who would listen. On returning from the UK and joining the TM CDC, Qu was disappointed to be appointed as head of a hotel inspection team. Rong, a fifty-something sanitation inspector with decades of experience who had previously led that team, respectfully stood back and watched as Qu bossed both the team and the clients around, a process that often ended in Rong having to step in to assuage irritated clients. This result in turn greatly irritated Qu.

Qu complained bitterly to me about a system that still ran on *guanxi*. While waiting for a driver to pick us up one day, for example, Qu grumbled about how late the driver was in arriving and how the driver's expectation that Qu should build good *guanxi* with him in exchange for his doing his job was due not so much to Confucian *renqing* ethics but to a lack of what Weber (2002) would call a Protestant work ethic. Qu told me,

> Chinese people are not *renzhen* [hard-working, earnest]. Like, I told the driver a long time ago to meet us here and at this time, but they are always late; we

always have to wait. It's not like in the United States where people say they're going to do something and then they do it, or if they don't, you can complain—here you can't scold anyone because you have to maintain good feelings—this is most important—if you scold someone you're only going to hurt yourself and not solve the problem because then people will be really uncooperative. This is a terrible way of doing things.

Qu's strategy to convince subordinates to act responsibly may well have been ineffective in any context. But here Qu's refusal to build *guanxi* became an ethical problem. He attempted to enforce a hierarchy that gave him higher status because of his higher level of education without engaging in the rituals of interpersonal engagement that had previously held such hierarchies together. This created ill will and also proved ineffective.

Although Dr. Rong and his colleagues grumbled about the "attitudes of 'young people'" (*nianqingren de taidu*) like Dr. Qu, at the same time they seemed resigned to their new positions in the *danwei*. Dr. Hong, a parasitologist who loved to tell stories of her hardships fighting malaria in the 1980s (see Chapter One), told me that she was saddened but not surprised when she was passed over as head of a department in favor of a PhD researcher educated in the Netherlands. Dr. Wu shrugged when I asked him how he felt about the imminent "cancellation" of the restaurant inspection program as part of the CDCs' phase-out of *chuangshou* programs and his likely reassignment to a food poisoning investigation team led by a recent PhD graduate. "I think it's right—the CDC should be doing these things. And [the PhD team leader] is very smart," he told me.

When pressed, however, sanitation workers also quietly defended the value of their work, insisting that eliminating the public hygiene work they did would only serve to hurt the larger mission of improved disease control. A TM CDC vice director who was in charge of all of the public hygiene (*gonggong weisheng*) departments in the TM CDC agreed, telling me in an interview near the end of my fieldwork,

After SARS, infectious disease control developed more quickly all over the country, and especially in Tianmai, whereas the Five Hygienes [*wu da weisheng*, see Introduction] have gotten weaker. But actually the Five Hygienes are at the basis—that is, my work is even more fundamental than infectious diseases. If I do this part well, it will affect the later occurrence and control of infectious disease, like clean food and water affecting gastrointestinal disease. So, looking at it from this point of view, we should emphasize the Five Hygienes even more.[15]

Wu also argued that his and his fellow inspectors' *guanxi* skills and practical experience were more useful than the public health reformers gave them credit for. "Our *danwei* has a lot of really young, capable people," Wu told me. "We just do everyday work [*richang gongzuo*]. . . . But we've done it a long time, so we can help solve problems. . . . Like with SARS or the [2008 melamine] milk-tainting crisis, sometimes they ask for advice, and we can help—[collaborators] trust us because we are familiar, our *guanxi* is good."[16] When *guanxi* was good and *renqing* properly nurtured, Wu suggested, milk was perhaps less likely to be tainted.

Plenty of younger informants also acknowledged the value of older colleagues' experiences, at least under certain circumstances. They respected some, like Hong, whom they considered to not rely too much on banqueting, to have sharp minds, and to be dedicated to their work, even if they were not that well educated. These were the types of older colleagues who would perhaps be willing and able to contribute to a professional common. Making the implementation of disease control projects dependent on *guanxi*, however, was to them an unacceptable way to "do public health" (*zuo gonggong weisheng*)—no matter who was doing it.

Serving the Professional Common

The post-SARS focus on emergency response provided a strong outside justification for my younger informants' claims that *guanxi* was no longer an acceptable way to do public health. *Guanxi* was slow and inefficient. In contrast, emergency response had to be fast. It also had to be automatic. It could not be dependent on the interpersonal dynamics of the particular people involved or on prolonged banqueting procedures, for which there was often insufficient time. Because the people involved in any particular response could change depending on the nature of the emergency, where it showed up, and what areas it involved, effective emergency response also required the building and maintenance of trust between strangers—colleagues who could be depended on to react expeditiously, even if they had never met each other before. Trust had to be transferable and had to be dependent on the process and the institution—not on the specific person involved. Data had to be produced reliably and shared transparently. Global pressure also dramatically raised expectations for the amount and quality of data being produced and shared transnationally.

All of this would require both a new kind of process capable of organizing lower-level CDCs, hospitals, residents' committees, and other institutions to cooperate on a permanent basis and a new kind of professional mentality that would convince those at every level to rapidly respond to clear lines of power rather than to ephemeral and shifting webs. This was the dream of the *professional common*—the dream that public health in Tianmai would eventually consist only of scientifically minded professionals who would work together to serve the needs of the entire group faithfully, simply because that was what professionals did. A major assumption of this dream was that all professionals would be able to *trust* each other to serve the common regardless of personal ties; that is, underlying everything would be a new form of *professionalized trust*.

After SARS, both local and central governments took steps to try to realize this dream. One of the first things they did was to address the problem of *guanxi*-impeded emergency response by attempting to detach outbreak reporting from *guanxi* webs. Six months after the disappearance of SARS, the China CDC launched the China Information System for Disease Control and Prevention (CISDCP), which required that certain infectious diseases be immediately reported in an online system that funneled data directly to the MOH (see Zhang et al. 2012). Local laws passed in Tianmai demanded that all infectious disease outbreaks and all cases of unusual diseases found anywhere in Tianmai be reported immediately through the online system.[17] Rather than leaving it to local levels to negotiate with each other about how and when they would receive and pass on outbreak reports and what the content of those reports would be, under the online system the expectation was that all public health professionals would adhere to a single comprehensive set of rules.

The goal was to eliminate the kinds of reporting delays and omissions that plagued the early days of the SARS response. A department leader at the Guangdong Provincial CDC told me that online reporting was the biggest change in disease control that had emerged from SARS. "It used to be that a hospital would get a case of flu and would fill out a form and send it in one big paper report to the street level, which would then slowly pass it up to the district, and by the time it got to provincial level it's a month later, the patient has recovered, and the outbreak is over!" she told me. "Now it's totally different—it's all computerized. So there is one case of novel influenza, and everyone up to the national level knows by the next day."

Under the new system, hospitals, schools, and businesses were expected to report "epidemic situations" (*yiqing*) to the local district- or street-level CDC or *fangbao ke* (hospital-based disease control department) as soon as they happened. The receiving institution would then enter the information into the online system, and the lowest-level CDC would investigate the situation (*chuli yiqing*).[18] If an outbreak spread, or the disease could not be identified, the city CDC would assist the lower levels in investigating.[19] The system did not usually work as smoothly as the previously quoted interlocutor suggested, however. Lower-level institutions frequently betrayed the principle of professionalized trust by failing to report outbreaks or even to turn over general surveillance numbers. Without any *guanxi* rituals to convince them to cooperate on any given day, or any significant increase in funding to offset the extra effort needed to comply, there was little incentive to risk the loss of face (*diu mianzi*) that might result from reporting an outbreak occurring on one's own turf.

This did not surprise older TM CDC members schooled in *guanxi*. The problem, they explained to me, was the anonymous interaction that was expected to occur between the public health worker or other reporting party and the abstract professional common, via a faceless computer system. Without any interpersonal interaction undergirding this system, there was no *renqing* at stake, no face of the Other to consider. It was the opposite of the embodied shared experience of the banquet hall. In this context, they told me, one simply could not trust that participation would produce any sort of reciprocal benefit—or that it would not in fact produce harm for the participant (such as political repercussions). Worse, to establish a set of standardized expectations divorced from *renqing* seemed to instrumentalize the relationships that did exist to a degree that started to feel more like corruption. When banqueting and other *guanxi*-building activities did occur in the context of implementing the new system, the stripped-down interaction was devoid of the emotion that was supposed to fuel it. Banqueting and professional rituals were combined in ways that made the stated goals too obvious for comfort and also failed to accomplish them.

During the course of my fieldwork, for example, TM CDC leaders organized several conferences in which they directly addressed the fact that reporting procedures were not being followed, gave a forum for representatives of all participating institutions to express their frustrations, and then followed this up with *guanxi* rituals meant to smooth over these tense interactions by reaffirming the importance of the *renqing* that supposedly still lay beneath. At two conferences that I attended in which community health service centers, CDCs, and hospitals were asked to devote unpaid time to contribute to influenza and diarrheal disease surveillance systems, city leaders repeatedly laid out the procedures that were supposed to be followed and threatened penalties from the BOH should the relevant institutions continue to produce bad data or no data at all. City CDC and BOH leaders gave speeches criticizing the poor reporting compliance of lower-level CDCs and *fangbao ke*s and publicly shamed those who had been especially remiss. They shifted rapidly among direct threats, rationalist appeals to professional responsibility and scientific efficacy, and appeals to the ethical responsibilities associated with the existing *renqing* that had been built over the years among various members of the institutions involved.

At one such conference, after the leaders delivered threats and made appeals, the highest city leaders departed, and a remaining TM CDC leader announced that a forum for "expressing opinions" would now take place. He reiterated how important the surveillance project was, how important cooperation between the hospitals and the CDCs were, and how important it was that leaders at all levels prioritize the surveillance system as they would another SARS. He then opened the floor for comments.

I assumed that no one would dare speak openly to oppose what the leaders had said, but I was wrong. The representative of the *fangbao ke* of a participating hospital immediately stood up, reached for the microphone, and began complaining that he could not be expected to cooperate without any funding for the project. "Your demands just keep getting greater and greater!" he yelled, sending off a flurry of similar complaints. As more and more members of cooperating *danwei*s joined in, they demanded funding, personnel, and logistical support. The city CDC representatives nodded gravely, promising they would talk to BOH leaders about their demands. Finally the TM CDC leader cut them off: "OK, we've discussed this for a long time, now let's have a more relaxed discussion over dinner and karaoke tonight and enjoy the resort, and tomorrow morning we can keep discussing informally." The meeting ended with a banquet in which declarations of *renqing* and commitments to cooperate were renewed, but participants confessed that these efforts had largely failed to produce the desired result. The public health reformers' objective of enforcing an obligation to serve the professional common seemed to be floundering in the absence of service to familiar *guanxi* partners.

Those with whom I spoke at the lower levels either denied that they were not complying or blamed insufficient support for failing to produce the numbers requested. Certainly the unfunded mandate was a big part of the problem: Only the BOH had the power to back up the surveillance demands with additional funding, and the Bureau had provided little funding. Adding on new job responsibilities without providing additional compensation seemed unfair to many, including cooperating clinicians who saw hundreds of patients a day and whose cooperation in reporting diseases to their hospital *fangbao ke*s had always been precarious. Without any means of coaxing their clinical colleagues to comply with the new requirements, the *fangbao ke* leaders claimed, their hands were tied.

But many of my younger interlocutors had a different interpretation. Pointing to the huge amounts of time that their colleagues in cooperating institutions spent banqueting and the money they earned from sanitation inspections and *chuangshou* clinics, the new public health professionals insisted that their colleagues should in fact have the time and money to come up with the requested data. Rather, these informants attributed the failure to comply to the poor moral character of some of their colleagues, who privileged their own interests and that of their "friends" over the interests of the professional common.

For those born and bred on *guanxi*, however, something else was to blame. By giving their colleagues a forum to chime in, the city CDC and BOH leaders actually were showing they cared less, rather than more: Such a forum should not and would not be necessary in a well-cared for *guanxi* relationship, and the banqueting that directly followed it felt awkward and lacking in the usual rambunctiousness. By crudely establishing a direct link among demands, complaints and *guanxi* rituals, they had broken with *li* and transformed a meal among friends into a lavish banquet that looked an awful lot like bribery.

Quality Data and the Production of Truths

Even on the occasions when their colleagues did dutifully enter reports into the online surveillance system in a timely fashion, my younger informants still felt that the professional common was not being effectively served. This was because the *quality* of the data that were eventually reported, they told me, was quite poor. During SARS, the central Chinese government was shamed on the world stage for failing to report accurate case counts to WHO and other global health bodies. A big reason for this failure, interlocutors from both Tianmai and WHO told me, was that there was little in the way of accurate *internal* data being reported. Even if national-level leaders had wanted to share good information with international partners, they were limited in their ability to do so by the unwillingness of those at the lower levels of governance to cooperate. This was not a new problem: Data fabrication in local reporting of statistics has long been a frustration for those trying to navigate China's system of fragmented authoritarianism (see Blum 2007; Mason in press).

The aftermath of SARS did help to ameliorate this situation. "After 2003, because the effect of this was so big internationally, we finally started to report the numbers, to gradually walk toward the truth," one TM CDC member told me. Another explained, "In the past, if someone reported 8,000 malaria cases, I'm sure it was really well over 20,000. Now there are laws; if you don't report, it's not acceptable (*bubao buxing*)! So if they say it's 8,000, it's probably not more than 10,000." International pressure and cajoling from high-level leaders had convinced even those at the local levels to report somewhat more accurate numbers. For Tianmai's new public health professionals, however, the modest increase in accurate reporting that followed SARS did not go nearly far enough.

Xu Dan, an epidemiologist at the TM CDC, explained to me that even after SARS created pressure from all sides to improve the quality of public health statistics, *scientific truth* (as she referred to it in English) still was maddeningly hard to come by. When local partners did report, they would almost always report the numbers that they thought would please their immediate superiors and their specific *guanxi* partners. Occasionally these numbers more or less reflected the "truth," but very often there remained little relationship between what was reported and what was actually happening on the ground. Xu explained:

It's so frustrating because I know that what I'm producing is not the "real truth" [in English]. I do statistics, but they're not real statistics. I want scientific truth, but the lower levels don't care about science—they don't get it when I say if we compare hand, foot, and mouth disease between this year and last year, we need to know that they are always reporting, consistently, in both years. I know they [the statistics reported] are not the truth, so it's depressing, because I have to produce a report regardless, have to do this stuff; it's my job, and it's what the leaders expect. But I know it's not the truth, not science, nothing to do with reality, so "*meiyou yisi, dou meiyou yisi*" [it's meaningless, it's all meaningless].

The failure to report "scientific truth" was not only a matter of trying to save face, as was so often assumed by frustrated Western partners, or even of trying to avoid political repercussions. It also had much to do with *guanxi* ethics. The production of accurate data, like the production of all data, remained reliant on *guanxi* relationships, and these relationships established a difference between data that were "true" and data that were, as Susan Blum (2007) puts it, "correct" (see Mason in press). *Guanxi* partners often produced statistics that no one believed to be "true" but that everyone found to be "correct." "Correct" data fulfilled the expectations and demands of a *guanxi* relationship. For example, if a *guanxi* partner requested that you vaccinate 100 percent of children in your district, and you are able to vaccinate only 80 percent, then reporting a 100 percent vaccination rate would not be *true*, but it would be *correct*.

For many of my younger informants, however, "correct" was no longer good enough. They repeatedly asserted that truth should be based on how things "really were" and not on whatever people said they were. But at the time of my fieldwork in 2008 and 2009, winning a promotion and maintaining a stable network of "friends" continued to be based on people's ability to deliver data that were "correct" according to the rules of *guanxi* and *renqing*. The continuous frustrations that my informants articulated about their inability to sweep away what was correct to get at what was true—contrasted with multiple incentives to do the opposite—laid bare at least two flawed assumptions about science more generally: that a pure form of "truth" reflective of an objective "reality" exists somewhere waiting to be found and that this truth can be obtained independently from personal relationships.

For Xu and her peers, science was supposed to be neutral, unfeeling, and devoid of human impact; *guanxi* was inherently antithetical to science (Latour 1993). As numerous science studies scholars have pointed out, however, all science is necessarily created through a series of culturally informed, relationship-dependent, and all-too-human measurements, decisions, and perspectives; the "truth" is always multiple and contingent (Fleck 1979; Latour and Woolgar 1979; Shapin 1994; Franklin 1995; Hess 1995). What Xu's frustration reveals, then, is the way in which the Chinese case, in failing to produce what Xu would recognize as the "truth," nonetheless brings this truth about a lack of truths into sharp relief. Xu, however, saw instead a quintessentially Chinese failure. Certain that there did exist an objective truth waiting to be found, Xu blamed her colleagues for being unwilling or unable to provide her—and the professional common more broadly—with the tools necessary to find it.

Determined to solve this problem, a few of my younger interlocutors began directly confronting collaborators about their reporting of certain obvious untruths, in an attempt to convince them to amend their claims. This strategy nearly always backfired. Returning to the example of the measles vaccination campaign, I observed one such doomed effort when the TM CDC vaccination team was visiting a residents' committee head to gain her cooperation in the campaign. The committee head promised rather implausibly that she could vaccinate every single migrant child who lived in her housing complex, in spite of known difficulties in keeping track of migrants and their families. The vaccination department head from the TM CDC nodded agreeably: Though it was clear to all that this was impossible, the goal of the *guanxi* ritual—to gain the residents' committee's cooperation in carrying out the campaign and reporting "correct" statistics back—had been met.

Just as we were about to leave, however, Dr. Feng, a young man in his midtwenties on the city CDC team, abruptly challenged the committee leader's claim: "Isn't it possible that [migrant families] might be reporting only one or two children in a family, but really they have more that they are hiding in the bedroom? Then how could you know how many children the migrants really have?" he asked.[20] The woman, clearly taken aback at this violation of *guanxi*-based trust narrowed her eyes and said no, that was not possible. Feng persisted. "Really? It's not possible?" The woman stalked to her desk and removed a form from the local branch of the State Family Planning Commission, waving it in my colleague's face. "I can assure you it's not possible," she replied icily. The subject was dropped, and the department head rushed to reassure the woman that she knew she would work very hard to make sure the targets were met. At the banquet that followed, the department head made certain that Feng enthusiastically toasted those who would have to repair the relationship that he had threatened. The young man ended up drinking until he collapsed in the bathroom outside the banquet hall and had to be carried home.

Feng had threatened the *guanxi* ritual by trying to open the black box in which public health projects took place. For any given project, the procedures by which collaborating partners obtained the numbers they did were purposefully obscured. In fact, the nontransparency of the *guanxi* web was helpful in reaching campaign goals, because if city CDC leaders could not see how the numbers were produced, they could not verify that anything was *not* "true." Latour (1999) argues that black boxes are at the heart of scientific production; they reflect "the way scientific and technical work is made invisible by its own success. When a machine runs efficiently, when a matter of fact is settled, one need focus only on its inputs and outputs and not on its internal complexity" (304). To my young informants, however, the black boxes that *guanxi* produced were not the essence of science but the antithesis. Black boxes were precisely what needed to be broken down to reveal the "reality" within: a neutral reality that existed independently of human actions, a denetworked reality that science studies scholars would say does not exist but in which Tianmai's young public health professionals firmly believed.

To carry out any public health projects, however, my informants had to accept the numbers that the black box spit out and had to act as if they assumed that these numbers reflected what had actually been observed or completed—an assumption that Feng had refused to make. Although the older CDC members did not seem bothered by this disconnect, the younger ones found the obvious unreliability of the numbers immensely frustrating. They took the poor quality of the numbers as a personal affront to their status as scientists and an unethical rejection of their colleagues' obligation to serve the interests of the professional common.

Professionalized Trust and the Global Common

SARS made the production of truthful data in China an international concern, linking the service of a professional common within China to the service of a professional common more globally. And yet international organizations trying to obtain accurate data from China often had even less success than Xu did. WHO had little enforcement power, and other international organizations had even less. Because there ultimately was no way, as a foreign organization, to force local officials to release accurate information, foreigners working on public health projects in China had no choice but to rely on the same collection of methods that their Chinese counterparts relied on—but these methods tended to work even less well for non-Chinese. Most savvy global health organizations operating in China partook in at least some *yingchou* activities and used their *guanxi* networks to obtain promises of information in the same way that their Chinese colleagues did. But their *guanxi* networks rarely ran as deep, and their other powers of persuasion were limited.

Western health officials and scientists were for the most part aware of these problems. Few were under any illusions that they received "true" numbers in the way that Western scientists were used to thinking about it. But there was little they could do about this. According to a woman who worked with a large American health organization in Beijing, "We have to trust the local governments to do with it what they are supposed to do" because she had no access herself. "And we have to rely on MOH statistics, which are almost always too good to be true."

Although most international organizations working on global health projects in China felt they had no choice but to accept the fact that post-SARS statistics were still significantly lacking in accuracy, some did actively try to force their Chinese colleagues to behave in ways they thought were more responsible. Near the end of my fieldwork in 2009, I interviewed Lyla Wang, who helped to run the HIV program of a large international NGO in Beijing. The NGO's China headquarters occupied a chic, all-glass office space at the top of a mostly empty skyscraper in a corner of Beijing swarming with expatriate businesspeople and diplomats. "It is all imported from [the United States]—the furniture, the décor, even the layout," Lyla told me as she led me on a tour of the office. Lyla worked for years on other foreign and national-level disease control projects before coming to this NGO. Working here was refreshing, she told me, because she was able to learn new ways to address what had always bothered her about working on public health projects in China.

Lyla shared my young TM CDC informants' impatience with how things worked, nodding vigorously when I mentioned their frustrations with their inability to gain cooperation from colleagues and with the endless banqueting. She felt that local public health institutions were inherently corrupt, that professionalized trust with Chinese colleagues currently was not possible, and that more effective change could happen through outside pressure than through internal reform. She told me that her organization tried to exert pressure on Chinese colleagues to serve the professional common by piecing together the numbers and reports the organization received, matching them with what numbers they were expecting and what they knew about China or thought they knew about the local situation and then pushing the local CDCs to provide evidence for their numbers when she was not satisfied. The emphasis was on ensuring "results" above all else. Quoting Deng Xiaoping's famous mantra, Lyla told me that when it came to the HIV work her NGO funded, "It doesn't matter whether it's a black cat or a white cat, so long as it catches the mouse."

For example, Lyla's NGO had recently worked with local CDCs to conduct targeted HIV testing of high-risk sex workers who sold their wares on the street (whom she referred to in English as "streetwalkers"). The local CDCs had promptly turned over the promised data, but the fact that Lyla was never able to enter the black box where the numbers were produced made it extremely difficult to tell where the data she received were coming from. She had no way of knowing, for example, whether the local people at the bottom of the *guanxi* chain were really testing streetwalkers or whether they were testing another group that they recorded as streetwalkers. "It's a good idea that is not working at all," a colleague of Lyla's who worked at UNAIDS told me. "When [local CDCs] needed to produce statistics for [the NGO], they just added the HIV test to the physical exams that they do at local restaurants or . . . at a factory. Then they reported those numbers."

Lyla acknowledged that this sort of subterfuge was a problem, but she insisted that her NGO had found a solution. She told me that when she suspected that statistics were not accurate, she confronted the local institutions with other statistics that suggested that they had not really been testing the target population. When they came back with statistics showing a surprisingly low level of HIV prevalence among the streetwalkers, for example, the NGO's workers noted that the reported syphilis prevalence was also very low and used these data to do something similar to what Feng had done: openly challenge the numbers that they were convinced could not be true. "If the syphilis rate is very low, that means they just mobilized the general population [not sex workers, known to have high rates of syphilis]. . . . So they cannot tell a lie," Wang explained. If she encountered the same backlash as the unfortunate Feng, she did not let on: The funding dollars and prestige that her foreign NGO provided may have shielded her from the worst of a slighted *guanxi* partner's wrath. Still, at the time of our interview, Wang was still waiting for more accurate statistics to be turned over.

In addition to challenging the black box statistics, Wang's organization also challenged the *guanxi* system of collaboration by attempting to use *competition* between *danwei*s in place of *guanxi* to force cooperation on funded projects. Wang said she would talk with the leaders of two hospitals, for example, and challenge each of them to work with the local CDCs on a project, with financial rewards promised for the most effective collaboration. Whereas my informants tried to cajole, shame, and reason with people to get them to accept a responsibility to serve the professional common, Lyla Wang tried to use the principles of free market competition. Neither party seemed to be having much success in dislodging *guanxi* from its continuing position of dominance, however—or in producing the ever-elusive "scientific truth."

Black Cats and White Cats

The assumption that undergirded all of the creative attempts to increase reporting compliance and improve accuracy in China's public health system was that Chinese professionals could not be trusted and that ever more intricate rituals of bureaucratic verification were necessary to get at the "truth." An ongoing suspicion that the numbers received at each point in the process were fake or incomplete threw the rituals of bureaucracy and of *guanxi* into an endless cycle in which both were constantly checked for efficacy and found to be lacking.

As we saw earlier, however, the purpose of *guanxi* was never to produce scientific truth. The purpose was to build trust between people—based in principles of *renqing* and sealed with emotion (*ganqing*)—which ultimately could allow things to get done. The question we might instead ask, then, is what were the attempts to replace *guanxi* relationships with a professional common actually getting done? Or, to return to Lyla Wang and Deng Xiaoping's formulation, what mouse were they catching and why?

One mouse that they were catching relatively effectively was the production of at least somewhat more accurate statistics about the prevalence of certain high-profile diseases and the dissemination of these numbers to a wider community of professionals. In addition, pressure from the new recruits did make progress toward decreasing the number of banquets that public health professionals were convening. And yet, despite these apparent advances, as of 2009 little progress had been made toward professionalized trust. Instead, both older and younger public health professionals told me that trust within the public health system had if anything *decreased* in the time since SARS. The new public health professionals were actively weakening older forms of community and trust before new forms were ready to replace them. The result was that both the older and younger generations of public health professionals were left with growing feelings of frustration, disillusionment, and unease.

Trust between public health professionals and local populations saw even less progress. This is probably due to the fact that almost none of the public health professionals I knew were making a serious attempt to build trust in this space. Even as they worked very hopefully toward a system of professionalized trust, and even as they criticized each other for failing to build this new kind of trust, few of my interlocutors ever committed to addressing their own roles in the broader problem of social trust in Chinese society. This was in part because of the continued tight control that the central government exercised over the sharing of data with the Chinese public and also in part because of a strong conviction, encouraged by state propaganda and shared between older and younger public health workers alike, that the general population was inherently incapable of responsibly handling sensitive health data. Whereas one informant told me that SARS created the idea of a "right to know" (*zhiqingquan*) and that the TM CDC announced "everything right away" to the public in the case of an outbreak, others told me—and I frequently observed—that only the most basic information about outbreaks was released to the public. My interlocutors told me they simply could not afford to risk providing the entire population with information that a good portion of it probably could not handle. As in their other dealings with Tianmai's largely migrant population, their goal was to keep what they regarded as a dangerous population under control. Releasing sensitive information would decrease, rather than increase, this control and could spark an incident of "chaos" (*luan*) that might harm the civilized immigrant common they sought to protect (see Chapter One) or further inhibit the development of the professional common.

Xu Dan explained the reasoning in this way:

> After SARS, because China already swallowed that bitter pill, discovered that concealing an outbreak, or using administrative means to suppress it, was a stupid thing to do. . . . Now our epidemics are open [*gongkai*]. But that doesn't mean we don't still write "internal documents." Why? Because we don't want to cause too big of a panic. The general public, they don't understand, [be-cause] China's average educational level is low. If you want to release it to the media, this will cause big social instability [*huoluan*]. So this kind of democracy, we don't want.

Xu acknowledged that the public probably knew that the CDC was keeping information from them, but she also saw no way around this. Building trust with her colleagues was her first order of business. Trust with the population would have to await an improvement in the "quality" of the population's members. Once again, service and governance were bifurcated: Xu's goal was to serve the professional common, while governing the general population.

One source of the difficulty that Tianmai's public health professionals met in trying to establish trust even among the highest *suzhi*, most highly educated members of the professional common, however, lay in the over-abundance of faith that they placed in the principles of modernity (Ferguson 1999). The critique of *guanxi* was based in an idealized vision of how my interlocutors imagined "modern" professionals should operate. This was a vision, however, that skipped over the linkages that exist in any society between interpersonal relationships and generalized rules (Giddens 1990; Shapin 1994). In attempting to force an epochal shift in which everyone would perform his or her duties according to a set of standards or rules inde-pendently of personal dynamics, public health reformers not only were try-ing to reinvent how public health works in China but were trying to reinvent how any professional community functions anywhere.

It should be unsurprising to anyone who has depended on personal con-nections to establish a collaboration with colleagues in the American or European context that the assault in Tianmai on both principles of *guanxi* and on principles of seniority did not yield the desired results. Professional responsibility and social obligation are everywhere deeply dependent on interpersonal ties and the intersubjective responsibilities that come with them. The attempt to push a depersonalized responsibility to "act scientifically" made little sense in the context of existing ethical frameworks and may have been undermining my informants' ability to build a cohesive professional common capable of mutual trust.

Epilogue: Anticorruption and the Death Knell of Yingchou?

In 2010, the rituals of banqueting in Tianmai briefly ground to a halt when a series of high-profile fatal car crashes involving drunk-driving bureaucrats led to a national anti–drunk-driving campaign. Local government leaders made the prevention of drunk driving a "top priority" (*gaodu zhongshi*), threatening stiff fines or jail sentences for those who failed to comply. This changed the dynamics of banquets considerably, much to the chagrin of the most enthusiastic banqueters, who grumbled about the inferior atmosphere that developed after the law was passed. Heavy drinking did quickly resume among some, but drunk-driving laws continued to be enforced, and it became the norm for designated drivers to sit out the toasting at some banquets.

Then, in December 2012, on his first trip out of Beijing, newly appointed Chinese President Xi Jinping traveled to Tianmai to honor Deng Xiaoping's legacy. He brought with him a sharp anticorruption message: The enrichment and entertainment of local officials at the expense of the public had to stop. When I returned to the TM CDC for another follow-up visit in August 2014, banqueting among local officials had gone partially underground. Public health professionals could no longer openly use public money to "entertain guests" (*jiedai keren*). Fearful of being seen engaging in illegal or quasi-legal activities, local government workers began entertaining in private eating establishments operating out of unmarked residences inside middle-class *xiaoqu*s, in a kind of Prohibition-era saloonlike atmosphere. The banquet that my CDC friends held in honor of my return fieldwork trip in 2014—which on previous visits had been an alcohol-laden raucous affair—was downgraded to a staid and quiet lunch in a brightly lit restaurant over a few dishes of food and a single bottle of wine. Banqueting and *guanxi* had not disappeared, but they might not ever be the same again.

One informant who had since my departure in 2009 transferred from the CDC to work at the local BOH—an institution known for its nearly constant intensive banqueting—told me in 2014 that the banqueting ban had made it impossible to make progress on any BOH projects. "We just *kai hui* (have meetings) all day long," he told me. "It's very frustrating!" So far, however, most TM CDC members seem to be taking the changes in stride. My younger informants, delighted at the lessened pressure to engage in *yingchou*, declared partial victory over *guanxi*. They told me that sometimes—not always, but sometimes—they were in fact able to "just send a fax" to their colleagues when they wanted to get something done. The professional common was starting to come into its own. It may have come via state fiat rather than reasoned argument or professional morals, but a victory was a victory all the same.

Chapter Three

Scientific Imaginaries

It was a smoggy Wednesday in July 2009, and I was in the maternity ward of a hospital in Tianmai. Three women were lined up on matching hospital beds, in various stages of labor. One of them, the one we were waiting for, was very close to giving birth. We chatted with the nurses and periodically peered at the birth canal, waiting for the baby and the placenta—the part that Jiang Tingting was interested in—to emerge. Never did Jiang, a master's student in public health whose research I was shadowing, introduce us to the woman whose placenta she was about to sample and who was quietly grunting and laboring in the background. After the baby finally emerged, one nurse pulled aside the placenta, took out the syringe Jiang had left for her, drew some blood from the umbilical cord, and then cut off a piece of the placenta. Jiang slid the sample into a test tube and took the vial of blood, and we both walked out of the room. She never said a word to the woman, and the dazed new mother had no idea that Jiang had just done this.

In fact, none of the women who came to this hospital to give birth knew that they might be participating in a research study, but the nurses repeated this procedure for Jiang several times a day. Jiang told me:

We wanted to have the nurse just take a little extra blood when they take the [mother's and baby's] blood anyway. But the hospital refused because it worries that the women will want to know what the blood is going to be used for, and then they might get angry if they find out it's been taken and used for this sort of thing. So what we worked out is to take a piece of the placenta. This way they never know. We just need it to get the genes; it doesn't affect them at all. So we don't need to tell them, and that makes it much easier.

She went on:

I do a survey too, after the birth. I just put on this white coat and walk in and call them by name, and then I say I'm going to ask them some questions about their pregnancy. They think I'm associated with the hospital and that this is part of the treatment, so they never refuse. At the end I tell them to sign their names. No one reads the consent paragraph, which mentions the sample collection, and I don't point it out to them. We can't let people decline to participate because that will bias the data! It's much more scientific this way, just getting everyone to do it.

This chapter tells the story of public health research in Tianmai. It describes the troubling lengths to which Tianmai's public health professionals and students went in their attempts to serve—and, they hoped, to gain acceptance into—an imagined community of scientists that I call the *transnational scientific common*, or TSC (Anderson 1991; Cao and Suttmeier 2001; Fong 2010). My interlocutors sought to serve this common by providing it with access to a valuable commodity: the biological tissues, fluids, and data belonging to Tianmai's massive population. In this way, Tianmai's public health professionals hoped to transform the populations they governed from dangerous menaces into lucrative career opportunities.

In the minds of many of the ambitious young people I met at the TM CDC and similar institutions, the TSC was the most important common they could serve, and conducting and publishing scientific research, especially in collaboration with foreign scientists, was one of the primary means through which they sought professional and moral legitimacy. Serving and seeking inclusion in the TSC provided an opportunity to, as my interlocutors put it, "develop oneself" (*fazhan ziji*) (Fong 2010; Kipnis 2010). Dr. Ang, a woman in her midthirties who worked in the HIV/AIDS department, explained this principle to me as we ate lunch in a mostly empty TM CDC cafeteria just before the start of the Spring Festival (Lunar New Year) holiday.

Surprised to see her there so close to the holiday, I asked whether she would soon be heading home to Hebei province with her husband and young son. She shook her head—they had gone on without her. The week she had off for Spring Festival was her only chance the whole year to get away from her *richang gongzuo* (everyday work), so Ang had decided to skip the festivities this year to work on her *keti* (research project) proposal and an accompanying article.

I was surprised: Spring Festival was the most important holiday of the year, and the one occasion on which even most members of the floating population took off work and went home. But, as Ang pointed out, she was not the only TM CDC member who had decided to stay: Scattered around the cafeteria were several of her colleagues, mostly in their twenties or thirties, all eating rapidly as if in a great hurry to get back to the office or lab. Suddenly embarrassed that I was about to head out for a weeklong vacation myself, I suggested that perhaps the TM CDC needed to hire more people so they would not have to work so hard. Ang shook her head and laughed. "Actually, to tell you the truth, we have enough people," she told me. "It's just that everyone wants to do their own *keyan* [scientific research]. Because doing an individual research project is the only way to develop yourself [*fazhan ziji*]."[1]

Developing oneself through scientific research at the TM CDC brought with it greater career advancement, higher status, and higher salaries. Thanks to Director Lan's heavy investment in research infrastructure and support after SARS, the TM CDC offered more and better resources to carry out *keti*s than were available in many universities. The reward structure of the *danwei* also provided plenty of incentives to publish the resulting articles: Lan offered monetary rewards of up to 10,000 RMB (about $1,600) for any TM CDC member who published an article in an English-language journal.[2] Those who brought in foreign collaborations or grants were also amply rewarded. Under these circumstances, few of the scientifically trained newcomers to the TM CDC could resist the temptation to try their hand at a *keti*.

In fact, many of my interlocutors told me that they had joined the *danwei* expressly for the purpose of doing research. The public health work that comprised their *richang gongzuo*—running vaccination campaigns, issuing reports, and investigating outbreaks—simply became the background against which their research happened to take place. And so service and governance became bifurcated in yet another way: Tianmai's public health professionals governed the population so that they could serve the transnational scientific common.

Ke Jin, for example, a young woman with a master's degree in microbiology, told me that she decided to apply to work at the TM CDC because of the ways in which Lan leveraged the *danwei*'s governing duties to produce research opportunities:

> At a lot of CDCs, there's a *yiqing* [epidemic situation], and they just go out and *chuli* [deal with it], and that's it. But what I really like about Director Lan and Director He [her department head] is that in the *yiqing* they saw opportunity [*jihui*]. They would go deal with the problem, and at the same time they would think, "Oh, how can I get a paper out of this?" or "What can I invent and sell that would help us do this better? What *keti* can I apply to that's related? What research can I do on this topic?" They have really limber minds [*naozi feichang linghuo*].

Many of Ke's peers complained that, although the opportunities to conduct research were great, the *quality* of the research, like the quality of the surveillance data described in the last chapter, was poor. A major culprit, once again, was *guanxi*. The stories that colleagues who spent time abroad carried back to China juxtaposed a romanticized vision of the quality and integrity of Western science with a condemnation of *guanxi*-tainted science in China. Professor Luo, a former TM CDC employee and a researcher at a university in Guangzhou who previously spent several years in the United States as a postdoctoral fellow, told me:

> China's system is much less fair and objective. For example, in the United States, if you apply for an NIH [National Institutes of Health] grant, you'll get a specific number assigned—say, 84.5. If you have 84.5 and someone else has an 84, then you definitely are ranked ahead of them. It's very scientific, very objective. But here it's totally subjective . . . It's all *guanxi*—you have to drink with them and give them gifts, but even more than that it's whom you know. If you have no *guanxi*, there's no way to really compete with the established people who know everybody even if objectively your project is the most "excellent." So it's much less fair.

For those like Ang who listened eagerly to stories like Luo's, the TSC was an extension of the hoped-for professional common discussed in the previous chapter. Ang and her colleagues imagined that, within the TSC, everything they were trying to build had already been realized. In the TSC, responsibility and trust derived from one's professional status, not from one's specific personal relationships. Colleagues reliably fulfilled their responsibilities to others, collaborators predictably turned over "true" data, and everyone had the autonomy and the space to produce rational, fair, and innovative science not subject to the biases that marred the work they did in China. To be accepted into the TSC, then, was to reach the pinnacle of professional achievement.

Dr. Mai, a retired epidemiologist who spent several years studying and working in the UK, was one of my informants who spoke eloquently of the ethical and orderly environment he felt characterized research science in Europe. Underlying this environment, according to Mai, was a system of rule-based, codified research ethics that Western scientists closely followed. Mai argued that China would not produce high-quality science until Chinese scientists began properly following these codes. Procedures like informed consent and confidentiality would provide scaffolding on which to build a more modern science free of *guanxi*, he told me (Oakley and Cocking 2001; Beauchamp and Childress 2009). My interlocutors in Tianmai adopted these codes, which they referred to as "international standards," as best they could—but they often found that the realities of the Chinese research environment meant that sometimes they had to bend the rules in order to continue serving the common. They did so with the conviction that, on joining the TSC one day, they would finally be able to follow the rules the way their Western collaborators did.

But the fantasy of the incorruptible research scientist who always followed codified ethics procedures did not reflect the reality of how science was done in Europe or the United States. Politics, self-interest, and networking influenced the science of Westerners, just as they did Chinese science. Codified guidelines and research standards were just as malleable, uncertain, and at times ethically hollow in the very settings held up as beacons for Chinese researchers as Chinese researchers found them to be in their own environments. And, in both settings, populations appreciated primarily for their value as statistical data were vulnerable to exploitation. As with all of the commons that Tianmai's public health professionals sought to serve, the dream of the transnational scientific common was a fantasy.

Chinese public health research, therefore, should be viewed neither as an anomaly, nor as the poor imitation of a more perfected Western science that many of my informants considered it to be. On the contrary, in doing precisely what "international standards" demanded of them, Tianmai's public health researchers took these standards to their logical, if at times ethically murky, conclusions. The story of public health research in Tianmai thus offers a window not just into Chinese science but also into the deeply conflicted ethics of the international scientific community as a whole.

What Is Wrong (and Right) with Chinese Science

The romantic vision of international science to which Tianmai's public health professionals ascribed presented them with a fundamental dilemma: How does one enter an ideal scientific community with science that is less than ideal?

In describing this conundrum, my interlocutors frequently pointed to what they referred to as the "Nobel problem": At the time that I was conducting my fieldwork, no Chinese scientist working on Chinese soil had ever won a Nobel Prize (Cao 2004) (the first such prize was finally awarded in 2015 to Tu Youyou for her work on the antimalarial drug artemisinin). My informants told me that the Nobel problem resulted from the propensity of scientists working in China to produce biased, poor-quality data that was not "fresh" (*xinxian*). This was not just a problem of *guanxi* or lack of technical skill. The deeper problem was that Chinese scientists only knew how to copy, they told me—they did not know how to create.[3]

Although the TM CDC leadership offered annual "innovation" (*chuangxin*) awards to those who came up with the most interesting research or intervention projects, most of the research that TM CDC researchers did closely mirrored projects already done elsewhere, often providing data for the "Chinese version" of public health studies conducted abroad. One student I interviewed, for example, complained that her project on cancer risk factors was not "creative" (*chuangzaoxing*) because the survey that she used in the study was almost an exact replica of a survey that her advisor's schoolmate had used in the United States. Her advisor had, in consultation with his

American colleagues, made small changes—such as the inclusion of green tea as a potential cancer preventative—to accommodate the "different cultural environment" in China, as the student put it. The assumption on the part of both Chinese and foreign scientists working on this project and many others I observed was that "international standards" are Euro-American standards and "local variability" occurs in China. Therefore, doing a study in China on a globally ubiquitous health problem like cancer would *always* be local and never general (see Shapin 1998; Hayden 2000; Gieryn 2002).

This denial of Chinese science as a potential universal meant that Tianmai's public health professionals felt permanently marginalized, doomed to forever produce a derivative form of science. They provided the data for others to analyze, the bodies to produce the data, and the staffing to process those bodies (Hayden 2003; Crane 2013). Always in the periphery, following the rules that others had created to fit the specificities of their own populations, Tianmai's public health professionals told me they excelled only at creating imitations—the scientific equivalents of the Louis Vuitton knockoff. And yet they felt that this was what the TSC demanded of them, that this was how they were expected to serve.

Hu Ruoshi, a new recruit who was working with Lan on a study of racial differences in genetic predisposition to diabetes, presented an example of the frustrations afforded by this kind of mimetic science. Hu's study used a survey adapted from one that a colleague had used in the United States several years ago, but Hu felt that the results were necessarily less meaningful than those that might be obtained in the American context because of China's lack of racial diversity. Adopting the racial diversity questions in the survey with little apparent awareness of the fraught meanings behind their original context (Epstein 2007; Fullwiley 2007, 2008), Hu told me that she had found a collection of genetic differences between the Chinese population and the U.S. white population. Yet, although she also tried to follow the American model by studying racial disparities within China—taking as her racial minority groups the Hui (Chinese Muslim), Meng (Mongolian), and Zang (Tibetan) groups because they were "the most different from the Han" majority—she had not yet managed to obtain a statistically significant sample from those groups because few of these minorities ended up coming into the participating hospitals, and even fewer met the conditions for her study (see Mason 2015). Even if they had, Hu sighed, the study would still not be as good as those conducted in the United States because China's racial diversity was simply not *"fengfu"* (rich, fruitful) enough, she said. "Of course it would be better if we could do it as in the United States," she said, "but we don't have many white or black people here!" Lacking the racial diversity that she understood had come to define good population health research science, the Chinese version of genetic diabetes studies could be nothing more than a poor imitation.

What Hu did not consider was how the quality of her imitation may have had less to do with the "richness" of her research subject pool than it did with the fact that American scientists in particular had been able, from their very particular cultural environment, to determine what the standard questions to ask were in the first place. Putting aside for the moment controversies surrounding the definition of "race" as a biologically significant construct in scientific research (Epstein 2007; Fullwiley 2007; Montoya 2007; Pollock 2012), it is worth asking why a society that was at least 90 percent racially homogenous according to their own definitions (and nearly 100 percent homogenous according to the American category of the "Asian" race) was using race as a category for the study of diabetes (Dikotter 1992; Harrell 1995). Hu had a simple answer: Racial differences were a hot topic in diabetes research internationally, and she wanted to publish her research in a respected English-language journal. Accepting the terms of entrance into the TSC as being set in an American-dominated West, my informants felt stuck in the production of second-rate mimetic studies. To be seen as making a contribution, their science had to basically look like everyone else's but be slightly more "Chinese."

The one place my interlocutors felt they could contribute something new, the one area where they could really excel, was in the sheer *quantity* of research data they were capable of producing. They produced this quantity by transforming local populations into what Sunder Rajan (2006) calls "biocapital": a commodity that Chinese public health professionals provided to foreign partners in the form of biological samples and biostatistical data. The role that Chinese public health professionals took on in providing biocapital for transnational partnerships was somewhat different from that described in much of the literature on global health science, in which former colonizers enjoyed enhanced access to the bodies and biologies of the formerly colonized (Lowe 2006; Crane 2013). In the Chinese case, access to bodies and to specimens was carefully guarded by Chinese scientists, who alone had the ability, via their *guanxi* networks, to touch and test the sources of their data. And yet it is not clear that the risk for harm was any smaller in the Chinese case. From an ethical standpoint, collecting large volumes of data from local populations on behalf of a transnational common was an inherently tricky affair.

Chinese Science and Public Health Ethics

In her work on globalized clinical trials, Adriana Petryna (2005, 2009) describes how transnational researchers studying the safety and efficacy of experimental pharmaceuticals made use of a policy of "ethical variability" to obtain data that they would otherwise not be able to obtain. That is, they applied supposedly universal international ethical guidelines differently in different parts of the world, under the rationale that what might be unacceptable in some places would be acceptable in others.[4] The implication in Petryna's work is that this practice should be ethically troubling because it assumes that subjects in some locations should not necessarily have rights to the same protections as those residing in other locations.

As I will show in this chapter, there clearly was an element of ethical variability in the Chinese research context. At least three important features of global *public health* research, however, rendered the ethical problems at hand somewhat different from those associated with global *clinical* research. First, public health research (like all research that makes use of "Big Data") looks for broad patterns, whereas clinical drug trials look for specific effects. Thus, in public health contexts around the world, large amounts of data are often collected without researcher or subject necessarily knowing what it might later be used for. Second, unlike global clinical research trials, which make use of large numbers of bodies in resource-poor settings under the assumption that these bodies are capable of standing in for Western subjects, public health research takes as its object of concern the "population"—an aggregate entity that is defined by the specific locality or group of people it represents and thus by definition is *not* interchangeable with other populations elsewhere in the world.

Finally, there is no consensus, even in Western contexts, over what the components of public health ethics should be (see Kass 2001; Bayer and Fairchild 2004). Clinical biomedical ethics—as taught in Western contexts and formally adopted by my Chinese informants—have since the Nuremburg trials established values like autonomy and beneficence as core principles (cf. Beauchamp and Childress 2009). The most fundamental principles of public health research ethics, however, are currently up for debate even in the Euro-American contexts from which my informants were borrowing. The existence of this ongoing debate meant that there were no clear international standards for my informants to be following, and it was in fact in attempting to follow the letter of what they understood to be the law that their practices took on the appearance of variability.

Having no clear code of public health research ethics to follow, my informants dutifully attempted to mimic the only clear international ethical codes that *were* available—that is, the ethical codes for conducting clinical biomedical research. In the absence of a formalized tradition of research ethics native to China, China's Ministry of Health in the early 2000s began demanding that all biomedical research—including public health research—go through Western-style Institutional Review Board (IRB) approval and informed consent procedures (see Nie 2001; Kleinman 2010; Nie et al. 2010).[5] Most universities and health bureaus in large cities in China now have their own IRBs, modeled after the U.S. versions (PRC Ministry of Health 2009b). The MOH guidelines for biomedical research ethics also mirror those in the United States: The risks and benefits must be clearly explained, confidentiality must be protected, and consent must be given freely and must be written (PRC Ministry of Health 2009b).

According to Dr. Mai, who was helping the MOH in its efforts to develop a nationally consistent set of ethics procedures, adopting informed consent was part of an "updating" of ethics from a "traditional" Confucian system of paternalistic virtue ethics (Oakley and Cocking 2001). In an interview in Beijing in 2009, Mai told me, "Confucius says, what you would want, you can do to others . . . But that is certainly not the up-to-date ethical principles. So we are introducing the informed consent . . . it's not just if you think something is good you can do it to people, but you should get permission. And not only permission but informed consent."[6]

At the time of my research, however, few of the public health professionals I interviewed saw informed consent or IRB procedures as meaningful regulators of their research processes. At multiple public health institutions in Tianmai and Guangzhou, researchers uniformly told me that they "did not have to worry about" the IRB procedures because their supervisors who had good *guanxi* with the IRB members would just ask the IRB to sign off on the project and it inevitably would. Also, researchers were usually more concerned with obtaining the consent of *guanxi* partners to help with a study than with obtaining the consent of the patients themselves to participate—for it was the *guanxi* partners who could round up the necessary participants and take the necessary samples. At the same time, the pressure on public health professionals to obtain large volumes of data meant that asking for consent seemed counterproductive, as it could only serve to decrease the subject pool. The result was that public health researchers rarely actually sought either consent or permission to collect data from the populations they governed, instead often choosing to hide their research agendas.

These workarounds may seem on the surface to represent egregious violations of ethical codes—and yet my interlocutors' actions must be viewed in the context of an already flexible interpretation of global ethics promoted by their foreign collaborators. In attempting to turn themselves into legitimate scientific professionals worthy of entry into a transnational scientific common, Tianmai's public health professionals exaggerated and thus highlighted some of the more troubling ambiguities of that common's ethical codes.

The Great Migrant Study

When Xu Dan set out in early 2009 to implement a *keti* on the health of the floating population, she certainly did not intend to do anything that could be construed as unethical. Xu had a master's degree in epidemiology and at the time of my research had been working full-time leading research and surveillance programs at the TM CDC for several years while also pursuing part-time PhD studies at a university in Hong Kong. By doing good research at the TM CDC—by producing useful quality data as best she could within the confines of her imperfect context—Xu hoped she might win a chance to conduct postdoctoral research abroad, where, she told me, "people care about the truth." Going abroad would also give her daughter a chance to go to school in a place that valued meritocracy over *guanxi*, she told me, and that did not suffer from the corruption that she felt had overtaken not just the public health world but all of Chinese society. And it would provide the stability that she felt Chinese urban society sorely lacked.

To have the chance to do all of this, however, Xu Dan felt that she had to please Professor Smith, her Australian-born PhD advisor, who frequently collaborated on research projects with the TM CDC. Xu hoped that Smith might be willing to use her own *guanxi* to help Xu enter a postdoc program in Australia. In conducting her research at the TM CDC, therefore, Xu looked for ways to provide Smith with something that she, and the TSC more broadly, would find valuable. And in the "Big Data"-obsessed world of twenty-first-century public health research, there was little that was more valuable than an enormous data set drawn from an enormous population (Hay et al. 2013; Larson 2013).

When I met her in late 2008, Xu was in the process of organizing a massive study of thousands of migrant workers across the city, looking at the prevalence of certain diseases within the floating population and the rates at which members of this population frequented certain clinics. Xu told me that she had chosen to work on this program primarily because "migrants are big now . . . a lot of foreigners are very interested in this [floating population] problem."

Xu had arranged to take her research subjects from the same data pool that one of the district CDCs needed for a *keti* it was doing to examine exposure to toxins among migrant factory workers and that the TM CDC microbiology department needed for a *keti* it was doing on hepatitis prevalence. By combining all of these projects and framing them collectively as a local government initiative to improve the health of the floating population, Xu Dan would be able to gather an enormous amount of data. "What we're good at in China is that we can get a lot of data very fast," she explained. Professor Smith, who agreed that migrant health was a hot and underexplored topic but who had no hope of gaining access to data on thousands of floating migrants herself, was delighted to offer support and some funding for the project. The project became an official BOH directive framed as a migrant health initiative—the line between research and public health intervention becoming invisible or even intentionally obscured (Sankar 2004; Petryna 2009; Adams 2013).[7]

Despite what she told me about how much she disliked the use of *guanxi*, Xu recognized that the effective use of *guanxi* would be key to her project's success. She threw herself into working her connections. With the backing of the city BOH and the TM CDC leaders' *guanxi* ties, she was able to mobilize the lower-level CDCs and their subordinate health centers to in turn mobilize their own *guanxi* with factory bosses to secure access to migrant workers laboring at about a dozen factories throughout the city. The factory bosses were asked to round up sixty workers per factory. Compensation and rights to the results of the study were granted to the factory bosses, to encourage their participation, nurture existing *guanxi* relationships, and because, according to Xu Dan, "they'll want to know how many of their workers have certain risks or diseases."[8]

Comprehensive health information (including data on vaccination history, mental health status, and detailed medical and hospitalization history), along with logs of factory worker exposure to various toxins and blood from thousands of factory workers were collected, compiled, and analyzed. Labs at the TM CDC and the relevant district CDCs split up the blood samples to test for antibodies to hepatitis and other common infections, and the results were used for both Xu's and the microbiology department's seroprevalence studies. The factory bosses' handpicked "small team leaders" administered the surveys. For two weeks I accompanied Xu Dan; Dr. Bo, a young man with a PhD in epidemiology who was leading the toxicology arm of the study; and a small army of research assistants and nurses as they trained the small team leaders and administered the blood draws.

At each factory Dr. Bo and his assistants spent an hour with the small team leaders and factory bosses, explaining how the migrants should fill out each item on the toxin exposure log forms and the health status surveys. Xu Dan met with the factory bosses to ensure compliance and explain the timeline. The migrants themselves were rarely involved in these training sessions. At one factory, however, as we met in a conference room to discuss the surveys, the bell for lunchtime rang and the room grew silent as we watched a river of hundreds of men and women in blue uniforms run past our window, jockeying to be the first in line at the cafeteria. When the last of the migrants had passed, Xu turned to the factory boss and asked him to call in some workers, so that she could make sure that they understood the surveys. "Make sure they are workers with low cultural levels (*wenhua shuiping*)," Xu said. "I want to make sure even they can understand."

The factory boss was visibly uncomfortable with the way in which Xu had, at least temporarily, hailed individualized subjects out of the floating population that labored at his factory (Althusser 1971). But he had a relationship with Xu and her *danwei* leaders to uphold, and he agreed to send his assistant to round up workers from the cafeteria. And so, ten minutes later, two women in their midtwenties, looking small and frightened in their oversized blue uniforms, appeared at the door to the conference room. Xu smiled kindly at the women. She invited them in, pulled out chairs for them, and reassured them that they were not in trouble. They looked at the factory boss, who nodded. Xu handed them each a thick packet and then leaned in and began to explain—first you fill out your personal information on the top of the survey, she explained, then you sign here where it says you agree. She explained that they were to read the whole survey and fill it out as we watched. Xu peered over each of their shoulders in turn as they worked. Whenever they hesitated before checking a box, Xu read aloud the line in question and suggested possible answers. They nodded their heads in agreement with whatever Xu suggested. It took the migrants twenty-five minutes to finish the survey, and then they were dismissed. We gathered around and looked at the results. "You might have to explain the questions and suggest some answers like I did," Xu said. "Otherwise it might take too long for them to finish, or they might not do it correctly." The factory bosses reassured Xu that they would have no trouble administering the survey and agreed that Xu would return to pick up the surveys in a few weeks.

A week later, we returned to the factory with two nurses and a cooler to do the blood draws. The migrants were told that the blood draw was a health checkup (*tijian*) "service" that normally cost 300 RMB but that the TM CDC researchers were willing to provide for free. They lined up to participate without complaint, laughing and smiling as they waited in line. Several workers murmured that they were nervous about having their blood drawn. Their co-workers teased them mercilessly—"It's just a little blood!" A female factory boss who was overseeing the line chimed in, "The doctors are giving you a free checkup! You should be grateful!"[9] (See Figure 3.1.)

As we waited for our driver to arrive and take us back to the TM CDC after a blood draw at another factory, I asked Dr. Bo if he had ever encountered anyone who refused to participate in a study like this. He hastily said that yes, of course some of them refused—though he balked at recalling a particular incident when this actually occurred. As we sat uncomfortably contemplating this paradox, Bo's colleague from one of the street-level CDCs interjected, "But that is very normal [*hen zhengchang de*], it is normal for a certain percentage to refuse each time." With this, a question about individual agency was answered with a statistical norm, and the subjects that Xu had hailed quickly disappeared safely back into the "population" (Hacking 1990; Kohrman 2005). One need not worry about the fact that migrant workers organized by their boss to participate in a study had little freedom

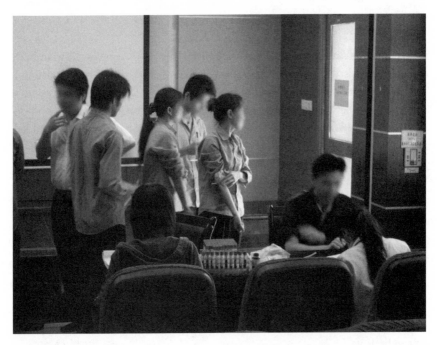

Figure 3.1. Migrant workers assigned to participate in the Great Migrant Study line up to have their blood drawn, 2009.
Photo by the author.

to refuse because what individual people could or could not decide to do was beside the point: What was important was that the population as a whole conformed to statistical norms—and the 90 to 95 percent participation rate that they were recording did just that. A commitment to uphold population-level statistics rendered individual-level agency irrelevant. The numbers had worked out somehow; it did not matter exactly how.

Just as it was normal for a percentage of the statistical population to refuse, Bo and his partner told me, it was also normal for the great majority to *not* refuse. In fact, the most important truths told by the statistics, according to Bo, was that the workers must, on average, be willing to comply. To explain this more positive side of statistical truths, Bo's partner produced a complementary truth about human behavior to help explain it. The migrants at this factory had been organized to donate blood (*xianxue*) the previous week, he told me. This meant that refusing a blood draw would be illogical—because giving a blood sample for a research study and donating blood were essentially "the same thing" (*yiyang de*).[10]

Dr. Bo, looking relieved, nodded emphatically and turned back to me: So you see, that is why we got the high compliance rate of fifty-eight participants out of sixty at this factory—you don't want to get sixty out of sixty anyway because that would be "*bu kekao de*" (unreliable) statistics—it's normal to *lou* (leave out) a few people, he explained, noting that two of the intended participants were out sick that day and so were recorded as declining to participate. Carefully following the form of foreign research requirements, Bo made sure that his team produced an acceptance rate that was impressively high but still statistically "normal" (Canguilhem 1991; Kohrman 2005). His ability to make subject coercion disappear revealed the depth of his knowledge of international norms: There was no coercion if the numbers looked normal.[11] But this faithful implementation of international standards also revealed the hollowness of the standards themselves: The attempt to produce the desired statistic became disconnected from any agency on the part of the counted subjects who refused to participate. And thus the researchers were able to tautologically prove the statistical truths that they assumed to be true in the first place.

What we are left with is a form of what Ian Hacking (1990) referred to as "statistical fatalism"—the idea that statistical truths, not politics or individual agency, compel the individuals who make up populations to behave in a certain way. An implicit faith in statistical fatalism in this case ensured that some people would be left out, even if no one was allowed to opt out. It also assumed that most people would opt in. The division of labor that Tianmai's public health professionals insisted on between those who were responsible for individuals (clinicians) and those who were responsible only for groups (public health professionals) precluded the need to consider the possibility that these assumptions might be false. Because they dealt only in populations and not in individuals, Dr. Bo and his colleagues did not need to draw any connection between statistical evidence of refusal and the capacity for individual refusal.

The statistical tautology threatened to fall apart, however, when I went with Dr. Bo to pick up the surveys a week later. To Bo's displeasure, we found that many of the participants had failed to fill out large sections of the survey or to sign their names on the informed consent line, producing a dismally low compliance rate. Bo scolded the small group leaders, who—grumbling that the floating population members' *suzhi* was not high enough for them to understand the intricate survey—quickly filled in the missing parts on most (though not all) of the forms, even signing the migrants' names for them if they had not done so themselves. Having been faced with possible evidence of individual refusal from a population presumed to be immune to the effects of individual agency, Bo and his colleagues moved quickly to erase this disconnect and restore their expected high-but-normal statistical truth.

When I delicately raised the question of migrant noncompliance on the car ride home, Bo's assistant attributed the problem to poor execution of *xuanchuan*, or propaganda. "It's all dependent on how well you do *xuanchuan* [propaganda] and how well the factory organizes it all—if the *xuanchuan* is good and they're well-educated in what's going on, then it's easier to do," he told me. Chinese and foreign translators usually translate the word *xuan-chuan* as "propaganda," but the word does not carry the negative connotations that it has in English, and a more faithful translation might be something closer to "information campaign." *Xuanchuan* used in public health campaigns usually consisted of posters or banners that promoted healthy or "civilized" (*wenming*) habits, provided information about how to recognize and care for a particular disease, or, in this case, explained the value of a research project and why participation was desirable. In the context of Xu's and Bo's project, *xuanchuan* alone was unlikely to have had much of an effect on persuading people to participate: For a member of the floating population living in a factory *danwei*, choosing not to participate in a project for which one has been selected was likely not an option.

But relying on *xuanchuan* for this particular study was problematic in another way as well. The sort of mass education that *xuanchuan* facilitated was intended to discipline a group to behave collectively in the *correct* way—to get everyone to stop spitting in the streets or to wash their hands (Foucault 1990). However, when it came to producing data that were not just correct but "true," *xuanchuan* was much less effective. Aside from the fact that *xu-anchuan*, in the words of several informants, simply "doesn't work anymore," here that method was unlikely to have produced Xu's "truth" even if *xuanchuan* relayed the information in precisely the way it was supposed to. That is because the success of Xu's surveys was entirely dependent on the collection of *individual* persons' data about their health, and training individuals to each fill out the survey according to his or her own conditions would require those individuals to learn, internalize, and use the information transmitted through *xuanchuan* according to their own specifications. That is, they would have to act as individual agents capable of making their own choices, at least when it came to checking boxes on a survey. In other words, teaching participants how to participate in a *keti* required teaching them how to tap into their own individuality—something that neither mass propaganda campaigns nor a public health profession determined to avoid engagement with individuals was designed to teach. Mere mass conformity would not produce the desired data because the statistics predicted that not everyone was the same.[12]

Whether due to a failure of *xuanchuan* or not, the migrant survey incident created an ethical problem for Xu Dan—although not in the way I had expected. When I went to her office to chat a few weeks after the study was to end, Xu complained that the factory bosses and the less-trained members of the CDC research team had failed to get the migrants to fill out all of the relevant parts of the survey. Nodding, I told her of how I had seen the small group leaders fill in some of the signatures and information in place of the migrants. Coming from my own academic "audit culture" (Strathern 2000a) in which the proper obtaining of informed consent was strictly policed and the forgery of signatures a serious legal and moral offense, I expected Xu to be horrified or at least embarrassed that the leaders had signed the consent forms on behalf of the workers. Instead, Xu sighed and said, "I know; they are so stupid! This is why the quality in China is so bad—they can't fill out the surveys for them! That will bias the data! Now I have to go back and redo the surveys."

The ethical problem that Xu identified here had nothing to do with consent. Instead, the problem was her inability to produce quality, "true" data—the same problem that characterized her surveillance work (see Chapter Two). Feeling unable to do anything about the poor scientific methods of her research partners but determined to rescue her project, Xu resigned herself to attempting to find the truth on her own. But, because of the huge sample pool she was using, she would have to rely at least in part on the data she had.

"I will redo the worst ones," she told me when I asked how she would find the time to readminister so many surveys herself. "The others I have to just use it anyway." What about the results of the study? Would they still be valid if she knew some of the surveys were forged, I asked? She sighed.

"No, of course not, but this is the only way we can do science here—I have to complete the project, so I will have to just use the data I have." Xu was under a great deal of pressure to generate data that she, her advisor, and Director Lan could all use to produce publications (and, she hoped, complete her PhD thesis). Xu's primary goal thus was to complete the study. Though she passionately believed in the possibility of a neutral scientific "truth," she also felt that pushing forward with what she had was her only option. To Xu, this was a different kind of failure in the production of truth than that exhibited by her Chinese colleagues in their (mis)reporting of disease incidence data: Whereas her colleagues, she felt, had acted out of moral failing, she had acted out of necessity.

The fact that she had to work with less than accurate numbers, however, implied that any potential attempts to apply the study to improve the health of the floating population would be based on data that were known to be inaccurate—a problem that Xu acknowledged but insisted she could do nothing about. Here is where the disconnect between population statistics and the individuals who made them up became particularly problematic: Whereas Bo's actions allowed for statistical truths to be preserved, the connection to individual lives had been lost. Xu would be able to deliver the desired statistics to her foreign collaborator and later to the TSC she sought to serve. But she would not be able to deliver any meaningful benefit to the floating population because her statistics did not correspond to any "reality" that the population might be experiencing. The data might be correct, but they would not be true.

This problem is not peculiar to China: One need look no further than recent data fabrication scandals in the United States to find evidence that what happened in Tianmai was likely far from a uniquely Chinese phenomenon (cf. Carey 2015; Foster 2015). Even short of data fabrication, Xu's project represents an exaggeration of the inherent difficulties involved in collecting data for any scientific research project, especially one involving a student or other researcher under great pressure to obtain results. Rothstein and Shoben (2013), Derksen (2000), Murphy (2001), and others note that there are dozens of types of errors and biases that make their way into any study performed by humans—including measurement error, ascertainment bias, participation bias, consent bias, and innumerable selection biases, among others. The case of the Great Migrant Study in Tianmai illustrates the human nature of all data gathering: What went on in Xu's case doubtless happens in more subtle ways in research sites around the world, and it is impossible to account for all biases adequately enough to render their influence null. The biases introduced in Xu's case, and her compromise—to work with what she had as best she could, while also recognizing the ways in which the data were flawed—may seem especially problematic, but nonetheless are indicative of choices that scientists around the world regularly make. Xu's case simply lays this problem bare.

My informants' foreign collaborators also made their own ethical compromises. Some of these compromises came across very clearly in the nature of the relationships they built with their Chinese partners. In one presentation that several young researchers at the TM CDC made to an epidemiology professor visiting from a prestigious American university, for example, the researchers suggested a collaboration to study the effects of a certain heavy metal on floating population workers at a local electronics factory, emphasizing that they had access to many people with unusual poisoning injuries—an attractive proposition for a foreign researcher rarely privileged to see so many unusual disorders in one place. The professor stated that he was indeed intrigued by the wealth of research possibilities and agreed to consider the collaboration.

The foreign professor told me later that he often pursued collaborations in China because there were so many "interesting problems" there and because his partners were eager to cooperate and were able to follow through quickly. Beyond asking them to fill out informed consent forms and get approval from their local Institutional Review Boards, however, foreign collaborators tended to avoid getting involved with how my informants gained access to the bodies they needed. In the case discussed in the preceding paragraph, the toxicology professor toured the relevant factories but flew back to the United States before the study was to begin.

Here was an apparent example of professionalized trust gone awry: In trusting his Chinese colleagues—whom he did not know well and with whom he had not built much *guanxi*—to carry out the research that had been agreed on and to do so in an ethical fashion, he unwittingly paved the way for unethical acts to occur. But the story of the hapless foreign collaborator who naively trusts his Chinese colleagues is not really reflective of the reality of how professionalized trust operates across borders. Foreign collaborators did trust their Chinese colleagues to get things done—but they were rarely blind to the fact that ethics are variable and that "getting things done" in China might not mean the same thing as getting things done in the foreign scientist's home country. The question then becomes: To what extent is the foreign collaborator culpable for any resulting harm that might occur due to ethical violations made in their name?

In an interview that I conducted following the conclusion of the data-gathering phase of Xu Dan's study, Professor Smith explained why the answer to this question for many was "not at all." Smith felt it was not her place to get involved or express concern about how her Chinese collaborators were gathering their data, even as she acknowledged that their methods were likely not meeting the ethical standards that she might expect from a Western collaborator:

> I get all my information from Xu Dan—she knows everything, she is very savvy. . . . I don't know about her methods—people do things differently over there, they have their way of doing things, and that's how it works, and I try not to get involved. I have no business telling them to do it another way. Every place has their own way of doing things, and in the future we'll all be doing it China's way anyway—certainly it's better than anything [my country] can come up with.

I asked her what she meant by this last statement. She replied, "They've got it all—they've got the money—Tianmai is swimming in money. They've got the brains—incredibly smart people there. And they've got the access and energy to do these projects." Did she mean how today you might say you want to do a survey of 5,000 migrant workers, tomorrow you can have twenty people out there doing it, and the next week it's done? I asked. "Exactly!" she laughed. Leaning back in her chair, she continued,

> Xu Dan has access to way more manpower than I do, and she's a student! They're very good at that in China—of course we have to wait until I see the write-up and see how she actually did it—then I will judge if the methods are good. But . . . I never quite understand why they're doing what they're doing. Like Xu Dan told me, "Oh, we collected blood from all these migrants". I say, "OK—why?" She said, "I don't know yet; maybe we'll need it for something, and anyway now we have it." I'm like, "OK, whatever!" I've learned to just go along.

Professor Smith justified her lack of interest in the procedures by which her colleagues at the TM CDC interacted with the population and collected their data through a mixture of cultural relativism, essentialization of Chinese culture, and hype about impending Chinese world domination. "I have no right to impose my way of doing things," she seemed to be conveying to me, "and I could not do anything about it if I wanted to. China is becoming a world power, and I have to accept 'their' methods." In the meantime, Smith had access to data that she likely never would have been able to gain access to if Xu had actually followed the sorts of ethical procedures she attested in her paperwork to following—including obtaining informed consent from 5,000 migrant workers in only a few weeks. Her trust in Xu became her alibi: Xu was a professional deserving of trust, and to afford her anything less would constitute a form of cultural imperialism. Between her having spent at least a decade working with Chinese researchers, and the knowing looks she gave me, I found it hard to believe that Professor Smith had no idea how these projects were actually getting done. But no matter how much she knew, the informed consent forms provided her with all the information she felt was relevant. The forms had been filled out, the survey had been completed, the data had been produced, the statistical norms had been met. The population had been studied.

Petryna (2009) has shown how this "don't ask, don't tell" policy is also prevalent in global clinical trials. But blindness to patient–researcher interactions was perhaps easier to justify in the context of global public health research, where the sought-out effect was on the level of the population. The peculiarities of how individual people interacted with researchers on the other side of the world in public health studies became even less relevant to foreign researchers than in the case of clinical trials. In the latter, at least, individual bodies stood in for potential consumers of tested drugs, and therefore the behavior of individuals could be important to the project. When it came to population-based studies, on the other hand, it mattered little from the point of view of project goals how people became statistics.

As many other scholars have noted, the bureaucratic instrumentality of human subjects protections is not restricted to research conducted in so-called non-Western countries: The protection of human subjects in the United States is often seen as secondary to legal protections for the professionals conducting the research, for example, and the signing of consent forms, even absent any forgery, rarely represents a clear-cut case of an individual agent freely choosing to participate (see Kleinman 1998; Strathern 2000a, 2000b; Flory and Emanuel 2004; Henderson et al. 2007; Petryna 2009). What Xu's case reveals, then, is not so much ethical *variability* as an exaggeration of ethical *fallibility*. A set of ethical rules enforced by anonymous bureaucracies and implemented through professionalized trust must often coexist with ambitions, interests (Hayden 2003), and transnational pressures that push strongly in an entirely different direction. To expect ethical purity under these circumstances would be unrealistic anywhere. Although everyone on all sides of a transnational partnership might claim to be following the same set of rules, following these rules in a place like Tianmai renders clearer the rules' inherent weaknesses and the fallibilities of those who employ them.

The "Relatively High-Quality" Research Subject

When I met her in the fall of 2008, Jiang Tingting, the student who collected the placenta samples, was in her second year of a three-year master's degree program in molecular epidemiology at the public health school of a large university in Guangzhou—one of several feeder schools for the TM CDC. Graduating with this degree would give Jiang a leg up in gaining entrance to a strong local CDC such as the TM CDC.[13]

Jiang had agreed to let me accompany her as she collected her research data for the placenta project, which she and her advisor were doing in collaboration with several public health institutions in Tianmai in an effort to identify China-specific environmental, genetic, and lifestyle maternal risk factors for a variety of congenital disorders in infants. Jiang was working as part of a team that included several of her classmates. The team fanned out across several cities in the Pearl River Delta to collect thousands of samples and surveys from high-risk mothers—especially those of advanced maternal age, those who had disorders of their own that put them at risk, or those who gave birth early—as well as matching samples of low-risk women. Genetic samples were collected from the mother and baby at the moment of birth, and surveys on risk factors were administered a couple of days later. Jiang was responsible for collecting several hundred samples and surveys at a hospital in Tianmai, prepping the samples in the hospital's lab, and then shipping everything off to one of her classmates back at the university for analysis. Her advisor had planned several English-language publications that he expected would come out of this project, and Jiang hoped to use the data to write her thesis.

Jiang first took me to the nurse's station, where we exchanged friendly hellos. "I worked really hard to get the nurses' cooperation, bringing them gifts, sweets, money," she told me. "My advisor was able to use his *guanxi* with the hospital director to set up the research project here, but it is impossible to do anything without the cooperation of the nurses and doctors. So I had to work on that *guanxi* myself." We entered the medical records room behind the nurses' station. "See, they let me pull the chart of whatever patient I want, record their information, and then interview them. Then I just leave the nurses a labeled tube, and they take a sample for me." She pulled a white coat out of a supply closet—"This is so the patients will think I am a physician," she explained. Then she pulled the medical chart for a woman with diabetes. She carefully recorded all of the woman's personal information and medical history in her notebook, and then we put on scrubs and headed to the delivery room to collect the woman's placenta.

In a 2004 article on the difficulties of carrying out informed consent procedures in public health research settings, Sun Wenjie of the national China CDC pointed out many of the problems with implementing informed consent that I observed in watching both Jiang and Xu conduct research: Researchers often used the power of administrative decree to acquire consent, they allowed those in power such as village leaders or bosses to sign on behalf of peasants or migrants, they did not clearly explain the study, they allowed research subjects to assume that signing the form or participating in the research was not voluntary, or they did not give a viable way for people to consider the risks and benefits and take the option of refusing to participate. Sankar (2004) and Epstein (2007), in their studies of research in the United States, point to similar problems in U.S.-based clinical studies as well, often resulting from the thin line that divides research and intervention.

As universal as the difficulties of obtaining informed consent may be, however, researchers in China argued both in print and in conversations with me that it was more of a challenge in the Chinese context than it was in Western contexts. Sun (2004) argued that in practice it was particularly difficult to implement informed consent procedures in China, given the "paternalistic culture," the difficulty of obtaining thousands of peoples' consent in public health research settings, and—pointing to a lack of social trust—the fact that "some people have a doubting nature" (13). Although the Institute of Medicine has argued that informed consent requirements for certain public health studies should in fact be relaxed (IOM 2009), Sun insisted in his article that informed consent in Chinese public health projects was critically important, not least because more and more research subjects were likely to be like those in Jiang's study rather than like those in Xu's study. That is, they were likely to be relatively educated patients who perhaps *did* "know how to protect themselves" and were liable to ask questions:

> The main ethical basis for informed consent is principles of beneficence and autonomy. *At the present time, people's education level, cultural level keeps going up, ideas are changing, more and more people's consciousness of their rights are unceasingly strengthening.* They urgently demand the right to make decisions about how to deal with their own matters. (Sun 2004, 13; emphasis added)

Here Sun recognizes within the population-as-research-object a collection of agentive subjects, with ideas and consciousness of their own rights. But although Jiang and other researchers I knew recognized that populations—particularly the nonfloating populations being targeted in Jiang's study—*could* be broken down into a collection of agents, they actively worked to not allow this to happen. For Jiang, the lack of interpersonal interaction with the woman whose placenta we sampled was crucial. If we had been introduced, if we had conversed with her as we had the nurses, then the laboring woman would have become a subject with a history, a set of relationships, a family, and a community—and therefore would no longer simply be a statistical contributor to Jiang's population data. This was something that Jiang explicitly did not want: "I don't want to know about their lives," she told me. Like Bo in the migrant study, Jiang's priority was to protect the integrity of the statistical result. To ensure that individual decision making would not get in the way of producing desirable population-level statistics, the people behind the statistics had to remain in a state of aggregated anonymity. The problem with informed consent in the Chinese public health research context, therefore, was not so much that, as has been popularly portrayed, "Chinese people" value the collective over the individual but rather that researchers carefully ensured that they were not dealing with individuals at all.

In the research projects I observed, concerns about the demands that those with higher "cultural levels" (*wenhua shuiping*) might have, therefore, did not lead to a greater commitment to carry out informed consent procedures. In fact, somewhat to my surprise, many of the researchers I knew were no more willing to try to obtain consent in the case of more middle-class populations than in the case of the floating population. Instead, fears that those in the former group might well refuse to participate if given the chance only increased my informants' determination to not allow them to do so. If the patients were able to choose not to participate, Jiang and her classmates told me, the quality of the data they collected would be ruined because of the likelihood that many in Tianmai's large and growing pool of what she referred to as "relatively high-quality" (*suzhi bijiao gao*) patients would refuse, thus disproportionately excluding many people from the data pool.

The problem, as Jiang articulated it, was that, unlike the floating population, the relatively high-quality patients who gave birth in her hospital *were* "high-quality" enough to *not* buy into what Mai had called "traditional Confucian" approaches of unquestioning submission. Rather, they asked questions, tried to take control of their own care, and asserted their rights to protect themselves (Anagnost 1997, 2004; Ong 2006; Ong and Zhang 2008). On the other hand, they were not quite "high-quality" enough, Jiang told me, to understand why the research was important, why taking a blood or tissue sample from them or their babies would not be harmful, or why they should sacrifice to serve the TSC (Weed and McKeown 1998). Therefore even the higher-quality members of Tianmai's population(s) were not capable of responsibly handling "the truth" about what Jiang was doing.

For Jiang, the relatively higher quality of her research population also failed to grant its members inclusion in the civilized immigrant common. The civilized immigrant common that my informants in Chapter One were striving to protect constituted an ideal type made up of modern, truly high-quality empowered citizens who were capable of regulating their own bodies. Anyone who might find herself in a midtier public hospital having her placenta sampled was by definition not quite high-quality enough to be part of this immigrant dream.

Making sure that most of the relatively high-quality patients eligible for her study actually participated was critical for a student like Jiang, whose ability to earn her degree depended almost entirely on producing as much data as possible as quickly as possible. Even while still students, public health researchers thus learned a variety of techniques for how to maximize the perceived "truth" value of their data while limiting any interference with the ability to obtain that "truth" that the informed consent procedure might introduce. Again, there is nothing particularly remarkable about this: Like good scientists anywhere, they were trying to maximize the results and minimize the obstacles to getting those results. They were just going about accomplishing these goals in ways that made the associated ethical challenges more legible than they might have been in other settings.

The case of Yu Waiping provides another illustration. When I met her in the fall of 2008, Yu—a classmate of Jiang—was working sixteen-hour days trying to complete a study on colon cancer risk factors entirely by herself, with the hope that her participation might eventually win her a chance to study abroad. This undertaking involved administering thousands of surveys that inquired about a wide range of lifestyle and dietary risk factors, working with the nurses to collect associated tissue samples from 2,000 colon cancer sufferers and a matching group of 2,000 patients with benign polyps, and then personally testing the samples in the lab to look for genetic risk factors—all within a twelve-month period. Because her advisor, the aforementioned Professor Luo, had failed to win grant money for this study, Yu had no one helping her. The study itself was only going through at all because the surgeon who was collaborating with them had offered free access to his patients and the hospital dormitories, and some minimal help with funds, in exchange for access to the data that they produced.

While accompanying her as she did her surveys one afternoon, I asked Yu how she dealt with informed consent procedures. Seeming to anticipate that this was an issue that would concern me, Yu sighed and explained her obfuscation of the procedures, much as Jiang did, as being born of necessity:

> Once the doctor was on board, it was a simple matter because the patients had to cooperate with the famous surgeon whom they revered so much. I just tell them that the doctor said they have to do this study . . . I know that informed consent is emphasized in the United States, and I think it is important and definitely the best way to do things. But there is no way to do it here. There is no way they would understand if I sat there and read the script—it would frighten and confuse them. And Chinese people really don't like to sign their names to things, especially when they've provided all this personal information. They are afraid that you will take this information plus their signature and go apply for a credit card or withdraw money from their bank account. I always make sure to ask and get them to agree orally about the survey.[14]

For the blood . . . well, the nurses always just get an extra couple vials of blood when they are drawing blood on day two of their inpatient stay, as everyone gets blood drawn on day two. And they know what I need so they don't say anything to the patient, they just draw an extra couple of vials to give to me, and they hand it off to me later. But when I do the survey later, I make a point of telling patients that I'm also going to test their blood. So of course they know that I must have taken their blood at some point, and they can figure out how it happened. But if at the time of the blood draw we say, "We're going to take two extra vials of blood for an experiment," that would really frighten them, and they would probably refuse. So it's a matter of how you present it. In China, [patients] just wouldn't do it if we needed a signature; there would be no way to convince them, and then it would not be possible to do any research at all. So to be able to practically to do any research in China, you have to do it this way. It's just the way it is.

Yu's concerns about gaining access to difficult data sources are concerns that any public health researcher might have. Relative to colleagues in societies with stricter regulations about deception in research, however, Yu had both more pressure and more freedom to take whatever steps she felt she needed to take to maximize data volume while minimizing consent bias. Yu was well aware of Western guidelines for doing research, and she agreed with Mai and Sun's assertions that they ideally should be followed in China. But although she did her best to obtain some sort of oral consent, at least after the fact—compared with Jiang she was both better informed and more self-aware about following global ethical regulations—she also felt helpless to implement all of the guidelines. Feeling unable to overcome a broad lack of social trust in China, Yu paradoxically felt she needed to continue to deceive the patients—thus inadvertently confirming their fears. Yu and Jiang insisted that they were acting responsibly toward the research subjects: Nothing they did posed any real risk of bodily harm. But carrying out informed consent procedures as written would cause them to not be able to act responsibly toward their advisors and by extension to the TSC, which to them was both morally and practically more important. In this context, trying her best to make sure the participants at least knew they were participating in a study was the best that Yu felt she could do.

The potential of informed consent to introduce bias is not trivial. In 2009, the Institute of Medicine argued that consent bias—which refers to the skewing of results that could occur if the people who consent to take part in a research project systematically differ from those who refuse to take part— is a big enough problem to justify relaxing consent requirements in large, noninterventional population studies (IOM 2009; Rothstein and Shoben 2013).[15] The perceived difficulties of obtaining consent on a mass scale, along with the perceived lack of harm to participants in studies of population data, has lent support in Western settings to the idea that informed consent might not always make sense as a strict requirement in public health research. Although Western researchers might be unlikely to sanction a waiving of consent requirements for studies like the ones described in the preceding pages, for Jiang and Yu, sacrificing informed consent procedures to reduce biases seemed like the reasonable, responsible, and professional thing to do.

The Ethics of Public Health Research

Public health ethicists Weed and McKeown (1993) argue that, because public health research is not the same as basic science research, those who engage in it must take on a set of special responsibilities. In addition to accountability to both fellow scientists and the population having its data mined, these include a "commitment to social goods," namely the "application of scientific knowledge to improve the public's health through disease prevention and health promotion" (1805). They also point out, along with other scholars of public health ethics (Coughlin 2006), that scientific validity and quality are in themselves ethical obligations.

The tension between the ethics of scientific validity and the ethics of accountability to research subjects is reflected throughout the Chinese and English literature on public health ethics. Ethical guidelines for all human biomedical research studies in China, including public health studies, are drawn from "international norms" and refer explicitly to the Nuremberg code and the Helsinki Declaration (Wang 2003; Sun 2004; PRC Ministry of Health 2009b). As Sun (2004) points out, however, it is not always clear how those protocols would apply to public health research, especially research of the type that does not test any drugs or introduce any sizable medical risk to participants. In fact, public health research of the type most of my informants conducted—that is, epidemiological research that involved neither giving nor withholding treatment, and relatively noninvasive biological sampling of blood, phlegm, or tissue—usually introduced few of either the benefits or risks to individual patients that have made up much of ethical concerns associated with transnational clinical research (Petryna 2005, 2009; Datta and Kessell 2009).

At the same time, the sheer numbers of people involved made obtaining informed consent from each individual person especially difficult, and attempting to do so could in theory do harm by creating barriers to the creation of knowledge that might be used to help populations (Gostin 2002). Sun (2004), however, argues that the subordination of consent to quality is inherently unethical. "If because of failing to get informed consent you fail to get people to enter a study, this will affect the integrity of the data," he acknowledged. "Even in this kind of circumstance, you can't deny informed consent" (14).

Scholars of public health ethics in the United States, on the other hand, have suggested that the ethics that guide clinical encounters or clinical research cannot and should not be the same as those that guide public health measures, because, according to Bayer and Fairchild, "At the core of public health practice is to protect the common good" (2004, 488), whereas the core of the clinical encounter was the patient. It therefore did not make sense, for example, to establish individual autonomy as a primary guiding principle for public health ethics (Kass 2001). In keeping with this argument, my informants did not see why they should jeopardize the validity of their study and thus what they themselves referred to as a potential common good (*gongyi*), just to give individual patients the right to avoid filling out a survey and having extra blood drawn.

The example of an anonymous HIV blood-screening program in the UK illustrates how this common good principle plays out in a Western research context. The UK program has conducted HIV tests on residual blood samples of millions of patients since 1990, without seeking informed consent, partly under the premise that "the epidemiological quality and usefulness of the data collected by the programme might be compromised if each participant were asked to provide individual consent" (Datta and Kessell 2009, 107–108) and that more important "'harm to others' can be prevented by high-quality information about the spread of a serious disease" (108). The rationale behind this was that HIV/AIDS was a serious threat to the public's health, that seeking consent from millions of patients who had already given their blood was not feasible, and that little discernible harm came from collecting this information and entrusting it to responsible professionals (Oakley and Cocking 2001).

The Institute of Medicine took a similar position in a 2009 position paper, arguing for the loosening of consent requirements for the use of individual health data in population-level research (IOM 2009; Smith et al. 2012; Larson 2013). The use of data that have already been collected for other purposes can be of great value to disease surveillance efforts as well as to efforts to understand the efficacy of existing treatments, but, according to a 2013 article in the *Journal of the American Medical Association* supporting the IOM's position, "to benefit from these advances and others not yet imagined, overly burdensome oversight and consent rules for research processes must be avoided" (Larson 2013, 2444). The assumption here again is that mining this existing data will surely benefit the common good, and researchers can and should be trusted to use this information without asking.

All of this raises at least two important questions to which I have been returning throughout this book. The first is the question of who is included in the "common good"—in this case, who constitutes the "common" when one is conducting a research project on local populations for a transnational audience of scientists. If the common to be served differs in kind from the population to be researched, then the rationale that the good of the common should trump individual participants' rights and interests no longer holds water. As discussed in previous chapters, the imprecision of the aggregate-as-common opens the door more widely to the exploitation of those not included within its boundaries.

The second question deals with the problem of whether and how professionals can be trusted. The IOM and the UK government seem to subscribe to the assumptions that scientists are inherently trustworthy and that one should assume that they will assure that any trade-offs between benefits and sacrifices are fair. Jiang, Yu, and Xu all considered themselves—if not necessarily their colleagues—to be responsible, trustworthy professionals or professionals-in-training, and they saw little sacrifice in what they were asking research subjects to do. Though they were producing new data and not just mining existing data, as Jiang told me, when she took a piece of placenta, "It doesn't affect them at all." Xu similarly explained that when she took blood from a migrant worker, it rarely brought any bodily harm. They had evaluated the situation and decided that it was ethical to proceed—a decision that, as scientists worthy of trust, they felt they should have the right to make.

Mai told me that although this approach was consistent with Confucian virtue ethics—a system that depended on the judgment of virtuous practitioners to determine what was ethical—it was not consistent with the Western clinical bioethics that China was attempting to adopt. Again, however, context is important: Although making the kinds of decisions that Jiang, Yu, and Xu made might seem antithetical to *clinical* bioethics in Western contexts, it actually fit in more readily than Mai acknowledged in the Western public health context. In some ways, in fact, China represents a model environment in which to conduct public health research in the era of "Big Data": With its enormous population, government capable of gaining access to large volumes of data without the burden of consent, and tradition of virtue ethics, China's "way of doing things" may in fact, as Professor Smith suggested, represent a model for the rest of the world.

In addition to a Chinese way of doing things, Tianmai provided something else assumed to be critical to the ethical practice of public health research and yet lacking in most other places in China: the possibility of broad social anonymity. In the literature on public health ethics, the more anonymous the data, and the more disconnected they are from people who could be found and known to the researcher and to others, the more ethical it generally is considered to be to manipulate the data without constraint (Peckham and Hann 2009).

Again, HIV/AIDS provides a good example of this line of reasoning. HIV/AIDS is a reportable disease in both the United States and China. Similarly to the UK case, American public health researchers regularly gain access to records of population prevalence and incidence of HIV/AIDS to carry out studies without obtaining any kind of consent. Though controversies raged in the 1990s regarding the ethics of name-based HIV reporting (Bayer and Fairchild 2004), there has been little debate about the ethics of accessing de-identified disease prevalence records. If the dataset is large enough, and the people within the population it references are already unable to be identified, then IRBs usually exempt the study from ethical review. In other words, granting anonymity and deidentifying data seem to automatically reduce future researchers' ethical responsibilities to the people who have become folded into that anonymous number. In the United States, as in China, the point at which people melt into an abstract collective also appears to be the point at which they lose the right to say no.

Dr. Mai, however, felt that, in the Chinese context at least, mass anonymity was not the answer—on the contrary, individualized rights had to be strengthened. Insisting that adhering to "international standards" should mean a nearly universal adoption of informed consent procedures, even in public health studies, Mai suggested that this could be accomplished through better education of both researchers and patients. According to Mai, researchers did not follow informed consent procedures because they were insufficiently educated that they should not place the onus of ethical responsibility on the virtue of the professional. At the same time, the people who participated in research studies ended up getting exploited, he told me, because they were not educated about research studies and so they did not know how to ask the right questions or even know that it was possible to say no. Of course, in the cases I have described, many did not know that they were participating in a research project at all.

My informants feared that an education campaign of the type that Mai suggested would only end up making research harder to complete without addressing what they saw as a more fundamental problem: a lack of social trust, fueled by the insufficient *suzhi* of Tianmai's populations. Yu's patients, whether they understood the research or not, might be taught how to ask questions, but they were not likely to be willing to participate until they were able to trust that the researchers, in serving the common, would not harm them in the process. And researchers in turn were unlikely to be willing to let participants make their own decisions about whether to participate until they were able to trust the participants to understand the wisdom of sacrificing their comfort or bodily materials for the good of the TSC.

In compensating for this mutual social distrust, however, my informants repeatedly generated the conditions in which distrust between researcher and subject flourished in the first place. Though vulnerable groups' distrust of researchers is common throughout the world—one need only think of the ramifications of the infamous Tuskegee study in the American context—my informants in Tianmai and Guangzhou were not worried about trust from vulnerable groups, such as migrant factory workers, because it was easy to get *their* "consent" even without it (Brandt 1978). Rather, they were worried about less vulnerable, higher-*suzhi* people who may well feel empowered to say no. Allowing these people to exercise their agency—trusting in them to make a good decision—would also mean allowing for the possibility of refusal, which in turn would mean losing control over the statistical truths that Tianmai's public health professionals felt compelled to (re)produce. It might also mean recognizing them as part of a common to be served rather than a population to be managed. For my informants, there was a clear resolution to the tension between research quality and patient rights: If necessary, patient rights should be sacrificed for the good of research quality. This, though, just leads us back to problems of power and coercion and the reasons that informed consent became the backbone of Western bioethics in the first place.

Conclusion: Service and Research

Over ice cream at McDonald's one afternoon in the spring of 2009, Lili and Xiao Chen, two young women in their late twenties who had bachelor's degrees in preventive medicine, complained about the research craze that had overtaken the TM CDC in the last several years. Although both women had recently enrolled in part-time MPH programs in Hong Kong, they resented the pressure they felt to publish because they did not see what the point of doing so was. They had joined the TM CDC right after SARS, when they thought they would be rewarded with a lucrative lifelong government career that would not require them to return to school just to keep up. "I came here because I didn't *want* to stay in school," Lili told me. I asked them what they thought about the CDC's transition since then from a "*jiance danwei*" (testing/ inspection *danwei*) to a "*keyan danwei*" (research *danwei*)—a phrase that many had repeated to me during my fieldwork. Xiao Chen shook her head in disgust:

> We're not supposed to be a *keyan danwei*, we're supposed to be a *fuwu danwei* [service danwei], but it seems that more and more of our personnel and time and money and effort are spent on research. But we're not a university, and we shouldn't try to be one! The universities would probably laugh at us, a city-level service government institution trying to do research. And what for? What are we really accomplishing? So that we can publish some papers that have no effect? I don't feel that any of the research that goes on in our department really does anything . . . And, anyway, all the data are unreliable—so it's totally meaningless as far as I'm concerned!

I asked what they should be doing, if not research. "*Kongzhi jibing, richang gongzuo!* [control diseases, everyday work!]" they replied in unison. Lili added, "We shouldn't try to do research here. We will just end up being the '*xiao laopo*' [concubine, lesser wife] of the universities."

For Lili and Xiao Chen, CDC research was an imitation of an imitation. It was an attempt to do what the universities were doing, even as the universities attempted to do what those abroad were doing—leaving the CDC with the lowly status of concubine, ever further estranged from the original "authentic" model (Benjamin 1969).

During the course of my fieldwork I had frequent conversations in which I had to explain to my Chinese interlocutors that in the United States there was only one U.S. CDC, and that this dealt with national-level concerns. At the local level in the United States, I explained, public health institutions often were primarily concerned with tasks that my informants had tried to abandon after SARS—like sanitation inspections—or with those my informants felt incapable of completing, like health education projects in disadvantaged communities. As Lili and Xiao Chen suggested, American local public health institutions were mostly focused on service; although many urban institutions were involved in some way in scientific research, they did not attempt to mimic the research agenda of the national CDC. This seemed to terribly disappoint people. They could not believe the system they thought they were modeling could be concerned with such mundane things as sanitation. The reputation of the U.S. CDC as a powerful, high-tech research institution had convinced them otherwise (Carpenter 2010).

Their disappointment was understandable, given the educational backgrounds from which the post-SARS TM CDC employees largely came. Trained as scientists, most of the young people who came to local CDCs throughout the Pearl River Delta after SARS wanted to produce science and wanted to set themselves apart from the less well-educated technicians in their *danwei* by "using their brains" and "developing themselves." They did not usually see "everyday work" as a viable way to do that. But with their work so oriented toward the production of publications and research data for an idealized transnational scientific common, it was easy for the local population to become relevant primarily for its value as biocapital and for the needs of the people who made up that population to get lost. At the same time, it was easy for the TSC to take on a life of its own, producing and distributing more and more data and more and more studies without anyone stopping to think about how individual scientists, in China and elsewhere, might be gathering their data or why.

I hope I have made clear that this is a real danger everywhere and not just in China. The rush to gather and mine huge amounts of data (that is,

"Big Data") has collapsed the difference between research and service—both in China and around the world—and, when these two things become interchangeable, it is easy for the goals of the researcher to gain the upper hand. I am not suggesting here that public health professionals in China or elsewhere should not be conducting research, or that none of the researchers I met cared about the well-being of their research subjects. Research *can* open the door to more effectively understand and thus in theory better serve local populations. And when they did talk with individual subjects or think about them as full-fledged persons, the public health professionals I knew generally treated local people with respect and expressed concern for their welfare.

As Lisa Stevenson (2012) points out in her study of "anonymous care," however, there is great harm that can come with treating a population as a statistic and with failing to recognize it as made up of people embedded in relationships and communities—even if those treating them this way mean well. And, as scholars of science studies have long argued, there is also harm that can come with treating the TSC as a neutral, fact-producing entity, devoid of human desires, human subjectivity, or human fallibility (cf. Fleck 1979; Latour and Woolgar 1979). This harm can be compounded when self-development is pursued at the expense of recognizing that both the "population" and the "scientific community" are also composed of "selves."

The desires of foreign scientists aided in limiting the scope of my informants' moral projects. For although their global partners made demands about the statistics they produced, the paperwork for which they were accountable, and the language they used, they rarely demanded that Tianmai's public health professionals do anything to actively aid the people who made up the local populations in question. In fact, foreign researchers benefited from the fact that their Chinese collaborators were *not* focused on protecting local populations because in this way they could have easier, faster access to more biocapital with fewer restrictions than they could ever hope to have access to on their own. A larger question for public health ethics, then, which extends much beyond the Chinese case, is under which circumstances global public health research can, or should, be considered ethical in the first place.

Chapter Four

Pandemic Betrayals

May 6, 2009

Dr. Han, a driver, and I are sitting in traffic in a large white van, headed for a downtown hotel. Dr. Han leans over from the front seat and hands me a white coat, a mask, and a blurry fax from the Hong Kong Centre for Health Protection. I squint at the fax, trying to make it out. It is a letter notifying the TM CDC that Jane Jones, an American woman who had been on a flight traveling from Los Angeles to Hong Kong with a passenger who had a confirmed case of H1N1 influenza, had crossed the border into Tianmai. The fax then lists her passport number and suggests that the TM CDC "take its own measures" to deal with the situation.

We arrive at the hotel and put on our white coats and masks. Our colleagues from the district CDC are already waiting for us with a hotel manager. They go over the information we have: The American and two South Korean colleagues took a car to the border and then crossed and took a taxi here. We don't know what happened after that, or whom they may have come into contact with. We have this license plate number, the district CDC woman told us—can you see if she can tell us anything about the driver, the colleagues, the car, where they went? Dr. Han nods and gestures at me. Maybe the foreigner can.

We go out of the room with our masks and disinfection equipment and approach the elevator. Some guests waiting to go up to their rooms put tissues to their noses and mouths and start to back away. The hotel manager tries to reassure them: "It's nothing!" [*mei shi!*] Two more guests walk into the lobby, hesitate, and also cover their mouths. One approaches the front desk to ask what's going on; the other runs out of the lobby door, covering her face with a handkerchief.

We step out of the elevator and approach the American's room. A tanned and freckled white woman in her midforties with blond shoulder-length hair answers the door. I greet her in English, and she nods at us and says, "why don't you come in and sit down?"

We sit around a small table, with the American on the bed and Dr. Han and me in desk chairs. Dr. Han pushes the slip of paper with the flight and taxi information over to me, and I hand it to the American: "Were you on this flight from Los Angeles to Hong Kong?" The woman nods. I go through the checklist of symptoms on the form, the woman shaking her head again and again. Headache? Cough? Fever? We hand her a thermometer—under the arm, I explain—and she unbuttons the top two buttons of her blouse, places it in her armpit, and waits. One of the district CDC women comes in: They found the other people in the car. Han rushes out, instructing me to finish the interview and to tell the woman that, regardless of whether or not she has symptoms, she will have to go into quarantine. The woman watches Han leave, hands me the thermometer, and asks, "Should I be worried?"

I look down at the thermometer. Her temperature is 37.2, just below the 37.5 degree cut-off to become a suspect case. I hesitate. "Well, you are fine, I think—no symptoms." She nods. "But unfortunately you are probably going to be quarantined here for a while, just in case." "Here?" "Yes." "I can't go back to Hong Kong first?" "No, you can't go back." She bites her lip and breathes deeply, but she is calm. "Oh God, I reported myself to the Hong Kong people when I heard about the sick guy on the plane—I guess I shouldn't have done that . . ." I run through the rest of the questions on the list. No, she didn't leave the hotel. She had no other contacts other than the driver and her colleagues. She does not know who the driver was or where he is now.

Han returns and gestures at the American: "The car is going to come soon," she says. I tell the woman to get her things together. The fear on the woman's face turns to anger. "That's it? Aren't you going to do some sort of exam? Isn't someone going to make sure I'm OK?" I assure her that if she actually develops symptoms she will be taken to the hospital and treated. But then she seems concerned in a different way: "Are they going to do anything to me in the quarantine?" She implies something invasive. I repeat the question to Han, who shakes her head: "No, just fever checks—but if she gets symptoms, then obviously we'll take blood and nasal samples." I leave out the blood part: "No, they're just going to take your temperature, but if you get a fever or other symptoms, you'll be sent to the infectious disease hospital. And that's where they'll test you to see if you have H1N1."

For the six years since SARS mysteriously disappeared, the world had been waiting for another novel influenza-like microbe to emerge. For six years, Tianmai and other Pearl River Delta cities had been preparing for such an event, determined to prove that they had absorbed the lessons of SARS and could keep such a microbe at bay. And then, in mid-April of 2009, the first influenza pandemic in forty years finally arrived.[1]

In this chapter, I describe the TM CDC's response to the initial outbreak of H1N1 influenza, or "swine flu," as it unfolded in the spring and summer of 2009. I show how Tianmai's public health professionals drew on the lessons of SARS to mount what they thought would be a globally laudable, professional response to H1N1 that would prove their worthiness both as members of the civilized, modern world—a *global common*—as well as members of the world of public health officials devoted to controlling border-crossing diseases—a *global health common*. What happened during the early days of the pandemic, however, instead revealed the ways in which my informants' full admittance into either one of these commons remained elusive. The difficulties that Tianmai's public health professionals had in escaping their region's perceived status as a source, rather than a victim, of dangerous viruses; their use of disease control tactics that were portrayed abroad as excessive and unsophisticated; and their disappointment with the failure of their own leaders to act in the professional fashion that they had been trying to promote since SARS—all frustrated their ambitions and revealed hard truths about where they stood in relation to foreign conceptions of the common good.

To my interlocutors' disappointment, even after all of their professionalization efforts, many foreign members of the global health common still treated them less as colleagues and more as a subgroup of an unruly Chinese population—an entity permanently in need of governance, rather than one in need of service. On the flip side, Western health officials also did not recognize their own constituencies as populations that might need to be governed on behalf of a global common that could include China. The gulf between Chinese public health professionals' reactions to H1N1 and the reactions across the Pacific raises the question of what global partnership really means in the face of a pandemic, as well as what the "common good" can or should mean in the space where public health becomes global health.

A Western Pandemic

Despite decades of preparation, the appearance of H1N1 came as a surprise. It was a surprise not because of what it was or when it came but because of where it came from. "You know, we did all this stuff on H5N1 [avian influenza] as the next pandemic, and here we are and it's from North America . . . it's not what we thought," a U.S. CDC employee who was living in China during the H1N1 outbreak told me in an interview. The first cases of the new virus were identified in California; early investigations suggested that the virus may have had origins in or near an industrial pig farm in Mexico. This was unsettling to many Western scientists because North America was not supposed to have the conditions that fostered the emergence of new viruses, much less the kind of new virus that would cause a pandemic. That was an honor that was supposed to belong to places like Tianmai.

Although the origins of the SARS virus to this day have never been determined (Janies et al. 2008), scientists at the time implicated "wet markets"—markets common in the Pearl River Delta that sell fresh produce, meat, and live animals—in the 2003 epidemic's emergence. They attributed the virus first to civets (a mammal similar to the raccoon) and then to bats, both "traditional" animals sold in wet markets for consumption (Kan et al. 2005; Lau et al. 2005).[2] By eating these wild animals, urban Chinese were portrayed as transgressing the line between nature and culture and thus launching SARS (Shortridge 2003; Goudsmit 2004). As Mei Zhan (2005) argues, "The story of 'zoonotic origin' did not blame nature itself for the SARS outbreak; what went wrong was the Chinese people's uncanny affinity with the nonhuman and the wild" (37).

Western media and Western scholars also pointed to the juxtaposition of China's many "backyard farms" with modern cityscapes as presenting another kind of viral danger (Bingham and Hinchcliffe 2008; Wald 2008). Backyard farms—small-scale family holdings of chickens, pigs, and other livestock—were ubiquitous throughout Asia, and observers commonly described them in derisive terms familiar to any historian of epidemics (Markel 1997; Shah 2001). The farms were filthy, backward, and uncontrollable; they allowed for an unholy mixing of animals, humans, and waste; they were contrary to modern agricultural techniques; and they were inevitable breeders of disease. Having been blamed for repeated outbreaks of the deadly H5N1 avian influenza virus since 1997, backyard farms joined wet markets as emblematic symbols of China's backwardness. Of particular significance was the fact that with backyard farms the "farm-to-fork chain may be as short as a few meters" (WHO 2004)—implying an antimodern failure to separate the meat one eats from the live animal from which it derives (Levi-Strauss 1969; Douglas 2002). As with wet markets, the backward transgressions that occurred in backyard farms were seen as dangerously intermingling with the modern world in Chinese cities. In Priscilla Wald's formulation, "The 'primitive farms' of [the Pearl River Delta], like the 'primordial' spaces of African rainforests, temporalize the threat of emerging infections, proclaiming the danger of putting the past in (geographical) proximity to the present" (2008, 7–8). Like the floating population, backyard farms and wet markets were inherently polluting in their persistent transgression of the line between rural and urban, traditional and modern.

Though other discourses about the origins of avian flu existed—some scientists and activists blamed factory farms, for example (cf. Greger 2006; Otte 2006)—Tianmai's public health professionals interpreted the ubiquity of the backwardness discourse as a challenge to their city's proper place in the modern world and to their own place in a global common. Locating backward diseases outside of China's borders had been a key part of China's modernization project since the time of the Patriotic Health Campaigns in the 1950s (Rogaski 2004); locating them specifically outside Tianmai's borders had been a key part of that city's modernization project since the malaria epidemics of the early 1980s (see Chapter One). For my informants, the arrival of H1N1 from North America proved that the mission, at least in Tianmai, was finally complete. Their city was no longer a source of backward diseases: It was a modern destination.

Though viruses in theory respect no borders, in practice keeping viruses from crossing borders is exactly how infectious disease workers have long tried to contain them. From the point of view of Tianmai's public health professionals, the initial appearance of H1N1 inside the borders of North America placed a clear burden on their North American colleagues to take action. According to their understanding of the professional responsibilities that they thought were expected of *all* public health professionals around the world after SARS, my informants expected their American and Mexican colleagues to move quickly to do whatever was necessary to contain the virus as best they could, so that they would be able to serve and protect the global common. And, after all of their diligent post-SARS reforms, Tianmai's public health professionals believed that this global common now should include China. Taking at face value the principle of "we're all in it together" that served as a rallying cry for post-SARS pandemic preparedness (cf. Chan 2007; Mason 2010), my informants assumed that, in the context of global pandemic response, the determination of which group would sacrifice more on behalf of the common would depend on the circumstances of a particular outbreak. Thus it seemed to them that this time it was the United States and Mexico, rather than China, that should be charged with controlling their populations to contain the virus and prevent it from spreading beyond their borders.

As always, my informants based their understanding of what a good professional should do on a set of "international standards." WHO and U.S. preparedness plans drafted in the mid-2000s suggested that exit screening and other strict containment measures inside affected countries should be taken to stem the spread of a novel influenza virus to other countries and delay the onset of a pandemic (WHO 2005b; U.S. Homeland Security Council 2006). A 2005 WHO plan suggested that at "phase 5," on confirmation of large domestic outbreaks of a novel human influenza virus, affected countries should attempt to "exclude spread to other countries/regions" and "make massive efforts to contain or delay human-to-human virus transmission and the onset of a pandemic."[3] My interlocutors took these plans extremely seriously: as the leader of the global health common, WHO was supposed to be setting the rules for all of its members. As one Hong Kong flu specialist told me, "WHO is only a platform for communication. But on this side, in China, Hong Kong, Taiwan, they treat the WHO's suggestion as gold. And this is what WHO said."

But what the WHO plan said and what the organization did turned out not to be quite the same thing. The preparedness plans drafted in the wake of SARS were geared toward an anticipated pandemic of the much deadlier H5N1 virus, and from the WHO's perspective H1N1 had moved too quickly and was too benign to warrant the kind of response that was originally planned. By the time H1N1 was identified, the U.S. CDC declared that it was already too late to contain it. WHO concurred. Although it did not declare a pandemic until June 11, 2009, the agency decided almost immediately in April that "geographical containment was not feasible, leading [WHO] to call for mitigation" (Gostin 2009, 2376). The virus rapidly spread beyond North America; on May 1, the first case of H1N1 was confirmed in Hong Kong.

A Political Disease Is a Useful Disease

April 29, 2009

Xu Dan sends me a text message, inviting me to come have a chat in her office. As usual, she is surrounded by mountains of notices, surveys, and photos of her daughter. I glance at the pile as I sit down, catching the words for flu, quarantine, preparedness. I ask Xu if she thinks a pandemic is coming. She laughs: "I think we all hope that there will be a pandemic—it's good for us, really, Xiao Mei ['Little Mei,' my nickname] because it causes everyone and the government to pay attention to the CDC and to public health." But hadn't everyone been telling me all year that all this attention and money that the TM CDC already has is here because of SARS? Didn't they already get the outbreak they needed? Xu shakes her head and smiles. "Yes, the government really paid attention after SARS, but now it's been six years, and that extra money and attention has trailed off. So now we need another SARS."

By late April 2009, small sidebars began appearing in local Tianmai newspapers reporting that a new flu had been identified among sick children in California. Local newspapers and television stations reported that President Hu Jintao himself had declared the prevention of an outbreak in China to be of vital importance. On the day of the confirmation of the first Hong Kong case—in a Mexican tourist—flights were halted between Mexico and China. The Chinese Minister of Health gave directives for every level of CDC nationwide to track down and quarantine passengers who were on the same flight with the patient, to report and isolate all people with symptoms who had recently returned from Mexico or the United States, and to quarantine all contacts of such people for seven days. The goal was to prevent or at least slow the virus from entering China. One official at the national China

CDC later explained to me, "Once [WHO] raised the [preparedness] level from 3 to 5, China immediately change[d] H1N1 flu from category B to A. That means they are more restrictive; you have to quarantine all the patients and also all the contacts." CDCs throughout China almost immediately began mounting a rigorous response, but, as with any public health directive, the specific nature of each effort was highly localized. As one Beijing-based WHO representative told me, "The guidelines [the national level] gives are the minimal to do. But that doesn't mean the provinces and cities can't do more."

Tianmai's public health professionals wanted to do more. They had the PhDs in epidemiology, they had the expensive new equipment, and they had proximity to a critical border with Hong Kong. But for six years, they had not had a reason to use any of these things to their fullest potential. Some of my informants felt that the post-SARS enthusiasm for funding public health had begun to wane. H1N1 gave them an opportunity to finish the reforms that they had started. "Of course we want swine flu to come and a pandemic to break out," one young man who worked in the infectious disease department told me in the early days of the Hong Kong outbreak in May, calling H1N1 "a political disease." "Why? Not because we want people to die or suffer; that's not good. But because the system is not good, and we need the government to pay attention as they are doing now, to bring attention back and get the money and will to change the system."

SARS had opened doors because of the seriousness of the disease and because of the economic and political fallout that followed. H1N1, on the other hand, at first seemed to many that it might reopen some of these doors without presenting any of the real dangers of SARS. It did not kill at nearly the rate that SARS did, and it did not spur WHO to declare travel advisories, but it still could draw international attention to the prowess of Tianmai's new disease control system. It could draw national attention to the need to continue funding the CDC system and local attention to the benefits that come with professional collaboration. And it could give local public health professionals a chance to show off their capabilities without risking their own lives. In this way, though they normally expressed bitterness about "political diseases," many felt that the political nature of H1N1 was surely its most positive attribute.

Some of the scientists who had devoted their lives to studying the flu virus and had whiled away endless hours prior to the appearance of H1N1 doing rote surveillance and testing work on ordinary flu were also openly excited about the intellectual opportunities that the arrival of swine flu in Tianmai might present to them as public health professionals. One member of the microbiology lab with a PhD told me, "I really hope we get at least one case, just to *wanr* [play]." "Play?" I asked him. "Yeah, you know, *wanr yixia* [have a little fun], get a chance to make use of all of our preparations, make it worth it—otherwise it's all a waste of time [*bai zuo*]!"

Preventing even one case of H1N1 from making it into Tianmai, however, soon became the raison d'etre of the TM CDC. By displaying powerful pandemic preparedness capabilities that exceeded the demands of Beijing, my informants thought that they would show the world that they were responsible professionals and that the TM CDC was deserving of the CDC name. They would succeed where even the U.S. CDC had failed. They would stop a pandemic in its tracks.

As soon as the first case in Hong Kong was confirmed, the Tianmai Bureau of Health issued a notice declaring that the city CDC, in conjunction with the city's Quarantine Inspection and Control Bureau, had the responsibility of keeping the virus from crossing the border from Hong Kong into Tianmai—that is, of "defending the first line" (*di'yi xian*). Tianmai CDC leaders in turn issued a notice to all departments declaring that H1N1 prevention and containment was now the center's highest priority, and they called a rare centerwide meeting to review the initial steps to be taken. "Whether it's bird flu or swine flu, the same principles apply," Director Lan said at this meeting. He made it clear that this response was to be the culmination of the TM CDC's many years of preparation, that everything they were going to do was entirely in keeping with "international regulations," and that the continued development of the TM CDC's own reputation and that of its members depended on preventing H1N1 from taking hold in Tianmai.

As initial measures, TM CDC leaders barred all those assigned to the emergency response team from leaving Tianmai until further notice. A twenty-four-hour hotline was established to answer questions from concerned citizens. Disinfection equipment was prepared. The flu surveillance mechanisms that had been put in place after SARS were tightened, and lower-level CDCs were told to report any suspected cases immediately. The Tianmai media also took up the cause. Interviews with SARS hero Zhong Nanshan, a Pearl River Delta native and perhaps the most famous doctor in China, rehashed stories from Zhong's heroics in identifying and stopping

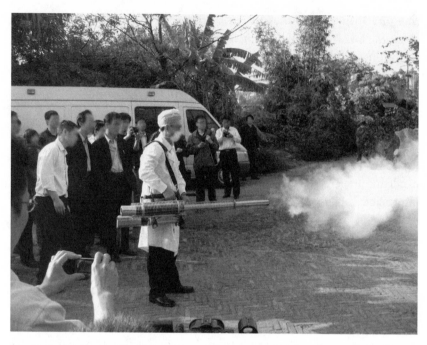

Figure 4.1. Public health professionals in Tianmai learning how to kill viruses with disinfectant at an emergency response training session, 2009.
Photo by the author.

SARS and offered up lessons for H1N1. A spread on the H1N1 threat in a local magazine declared, "From this H1N1 that was brought by North Americans, we can easily think back to the SARS panic six years ago. Actually today Chinese people remain in combative readiness for H1N1 and benefited from the life and death practice of six years ago" (Hong 2009, 35). (See Figure 4.1.)

The porous border with Hong Kong represented the frontlines of the H1N1 battle. The ambiguous status of Hong Kong—just foreign enough that its people could lawfully be kept out of the Mainland but just Chinese enough that they should rightfully be expected to cooperate fully in the task of protecting the motherland—established the former colony as both an asset and a threat to the flu prevention efforts of Tianmai and other Pearl River Delta cities. After SARS, Hong Kong's Centre for Health Protection (CHP) established official relations with the Guangdong provincial BOH, allowing the two institutions to report outbreaks to each other without having to go through Beijing. The CHP also developed closer relations with large city CDCs in Guangdong province, including the TM CDC, but these connections remained informal. As a courtesy, the CHP notified the TM CDC about any changes in its emergency response policies. In the early days of H1N1 the CHP also sent faxes to the TM CDC whenever a suspected case or contact crossed the border (no banqueting required!).

The CHP's ability to influence the actions of its counterparts in Guangdong remained limited, however. According to a CHP official whom I interviewed in July 2009, "Often Guangdong might want to follow us, but they have to wait for Beijing; they still have to do what Beijing says, so that's frustrating for them." Despite their proximity to Hong Kong, TM CDC leaders were mostly taking cues from local Mainland leaders—cues that in turn had their origins in Beijing. This fact bothered many of Tianmai's public health professionals, who felt that Hong Kong served as a more appropriate model for their response (MacPhail 2014).

On the other hand, with the arrival of H1N1, Hong Kong and its dense population also came to represent for Tianmai a holding pen of contagion, the boundaries of which had to be carefully patrolled. Whereas my informants in the past had seen the leakiness of the border as an opportunity for Tianmai to absorb more of Hong Kong's cosmopolitan reputation and economic opportunities, with H1N1 these same attributes also marked Hong Kong as a threat. The highly mobile population of Hong Kong, like the floating population, had become a "population problem" (*renkou wenti*).

For Tianmai's public health professionals, these two population problems became intertwined. Whereas the mobile Hong Kong population threatened to provide the spark for a domestic epidemic, the mobile floating population threatened to spread the fire. A department head at the Di'yi District CDC told me that, along these lines, "We have so many workers in Tianmai, crowded together in factories; just think, if the virus got loose in a factory, this would be big trouble. And these people don't go to the hospital when they're sick—they just spread it around without anyone knowing; it's very hard to control."

Because the floating population was so difficult to control, my informants told me, it became all the more essential to try to control the population crossing over the border. One of the first measures that the TM CDC implemented, in conjunction with the city Quarantine Bureau, was to require each person who crossed the border from Hong Kong and traveled into Tianmai to complete a health report attesting to his or her lack of flu symptoms and reporting where else he or she had traveled during the previous seven days. The goal of these efforts was to refine the fuzzy Mainland–Hong Kong border, and thus the boundary between infected and not-yet-infected populations, into something a little sharper, a little more concrete.

In service of this goal, the Tianmai Quarantine Bureau reassigned much of its personnel to staff flu prevention booths, where they examined health reports, pulled aside suspect travelers for interviews or exams, and pointed laser thermometers shaped like guns at the foreheads of anyone who had transited through Hong Kong from an "epidemic region"—at first defined as Texas, California, or Mexico, and later expanded to include Japan, the rest of the United States, Canada, and eventually Hong Kong itself. In keeping with TM BOH guidelines, anyone attempting to enter Tianmai from Hong Kong who reported recent travel to an epidemic region and showed a fever of at least 37.5 degrees or any other flulike symptoms would be taken to the designated swine flu hospital—an infectious disease hospital that had also been the receiving hospital for SARS patients—to be evaluated by TM CDC workers. Anyone still exhibiting symptoms at that point would be isolated until swine flu was ruled out through laboratory tests, or for seven days after cessation of flu symptoms. In addition, TM CDC workers detained anyone reporting contact with an H1N1 patient, or seated on an airplane with a suspected case, in a quarantine facility on the outskirts of Tianmai, where he or she would be monitored and treated with Tamiflu and Traditional Chinese Medicine (TCM) for seven days.

In the early days of the pandemic, the TM CDC sent investigators to the hospital whenever a suspected case was brought in. Later it sent workers to stay in dormitories at the hospital for two-week shifts, where they were on call twenty-four hours a day. The vast majority of the young people hired since SARS were pulled from their "everyday work" (*richang gongzuo*) and assigned to carry out these tasks. All other programs, including surveillance for other infectious diseases common in Tianmai in the spring and summer, were effectively put on hold.

At the beginning of the campaign, a wave of excitement rushed through the TM CDC. Midnight calls to don full-body biohazard suits in the searing heat and investigate the steady stream of suspected cases were met with enthusiasm. Eager young workers who had spent their entire short careers training for a moment like this volunteered to take up residence in the quar-

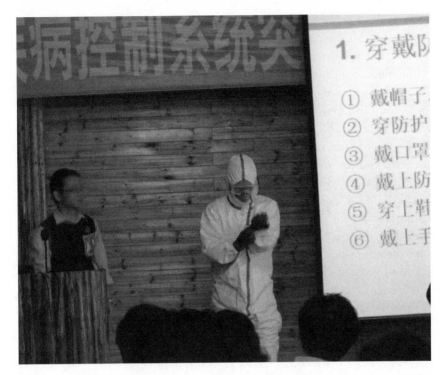

Figure 4.2. Public health professionals in Tianmai learn how to properly put on and take off a biohazard suit at an emergency response training session, 2009.
Photo by the author.

antine camp. Quarantine notices were issued with a sense of importance, and incensed foreign travelers were calmed with appeals to a moral high ground based on, as was explained to me, "the laws of our country and of the international community, internationally accepted regulations, and a responsibility to society and the world." When moral appeals did not work, promises of laptop computers, free mobile phones, and Western-style meals helped to soothe the quarantined travelers' unsteady nerves. The whole TM CDC bustled with excitement, a sense of purpose, and a feeling of pride that the people there were carrying out a rigorous, professional response worthy of the CDC name. The front pages of newspapers in Tianmai throughout the month of May were splashed with photographs of public health professionals in biohazard suits posing alongside grateful patients and articles recounting dramatic quarantine efforts taking place all over China. (See Figure 4.2.)

When the crisis first started, everyone at the TM CDC made a point of showing off the *danwei*'s high level of transparency and openness about H1N1. Their insistence on reporting every single suspect case, and their willingness to include me in their response, surprised and rather unnerved me. Influenza containment work was ordinarily considered to be highly "sensitive" (*mingan*), and in the past my informants at the TM CDC had strictly guarded information about isolated outbreaks of avian influenza in files stamped "top secret" (*juemi*). Therefore, although I immediately volunteered to help with the H1N1 testing and containment effort, I was surprised when, about a week after the arrival of the first case in Hong Kong, Huang Qing, a master's graduate in the TM CDC's epidemiology department, actually did call me for help. Hoping that I could act as an interpreter for a French patient, her colleagues picked me up late on a Tuesday night, brought me to the infectious disease hospital, helped me into a biohazard suit, and asked me to interview a patient who had just been brought in from the border. The next day, the usually tight-lipped leader of the infectious disease department called me, requesting that I serve as an interpreter for the American businesswoman who was sent off to quarantine. Thrilled with the high level of access I was achieving, I began making plans to spend the rest of my fieldwork working on the H1N1 containment effort.

But as abruptly as it began, my good fortune ended. Despite being praised as a "Tianmai CDC hero" and compared to the Canadian physician and Anti-Japanese War hero Norman Bethune for my help in successfully communicating calm and convincing messages to foreign patients in a time of crisis, the phone calls quickly stopped, and my hopes of eventually seeing the "most secret" (*zui baomi*) quarantine facility where all of the healthy contacts were being held were dashed. It was only much later that I found out that I had probably been called twice during that one twenty-four-hour period only out of desperation. The night that I was first called, a boat traveling from Hong Kong carrying forty-five passengers from an international flight was stopped due to a suspect case aboard, and all forty-five passengers were sent to the quarantine facility in Tianmai. Few could speak Chinese, and for the eighteen hours or so that they were held before H1N1 was ruled out, the Tianmai CDC system was desperately shorthanded for foreign-language speakers. I had only been given as much access as was absolutely necessary. I never was allowed to visit the quarantine facility during its three months of operation.

This outcome did not surprise me. Despite all of the increases in transparency after SARS, my interlocutors periodically reminded me that they knew exactly where the line was in terms of what they could tell a foreigner, and they were not about to cross that line and jeopardize their own careers on my behalf. They also knew where the line was in terms of disclosing information to the media or to the Chinese public. The head of the flu surveillance team explained that, although SARS had shifted the line, it was still very much intact—and for good reason. Drawing once again on the familiar tropes of stability and chaos that underlay so many of my informants' stories about their own professional ambitions and fears, Dr. Wang told me that, if ordinary Chinese people knew too much about H1N1, "They would start a panic (*konghuang*), and we really have to be careful about chaos (*huoluan*)" (see Chapter Two; also Mason in press).

Most of my TM CDC contacts continued to take a dimmer view, however, of the motivations of their colleagues at the lower levels in not reporting cases of H1N1 within the internal surveillance system. Dr. Peng told me in early May that she suspected that the fact that no cases of H1N1 had been reported yet in Tianmai had to do with a blatant disregard for professional responsibility on the part of her colleagues who, she suspected, were covering for their "friends" who were fearful of losing face if they reported the first case of H1N1. Peng told me with frustration that, even in an "emergency situation" like the H1N1 outbreak, concerns about *guanxi* and face still trumped concerns about professional responsibility and truth. A few weeks after we had this conversation, the first case of H1N1 was reported in Tianmai, suddenly opening the floodgates. Dozens of reports of suspect cases quickly poured in. Peng quipped, "See, they were all holding those cases, waiting for the symbolic first one."

Well before this first case arrived, the tone at the TM CDC had already begun to sour. During the SARS epidemic, China's leaders and public health professionals received international praise for implementing harsh but apparently successful control measures within their borders (Kaufman 2006; Saich 2006). In instituting similar measures in response to H1N1, however, Chinese public health professionals focused on controlling foreign travelers in an effort to contain the virus *outside* rather than *inside* China's borders—a distinction that they thought should not be important in light of persistent proclamations from WHO and other global health bodies that controlling pandemics was a collective responsibility of the global health common to protect an overall global common good. Instead, the same organizations that had praised China six years earlier for so effectively controlling its dangerous population balked when the definition of a dangerous population shifted to include foreign subjects not accustomed to being treated as an unindividuated aggregate of risk. In response to China's H1N1 control actions, WHO, CDC, and others this time offered only tepid support and eventually gentle criticism, calling the response an overreaction. Meanwhile, Western news outlets flung accusations of xenophobia and published harrowing accounts of tourists' quarantine experiences in allegedly backward conditions at the hands of a draconian state (Metzl 2009; Stolberg and Robinson 2009).

The effect was to build, rather than tear down, borders between WHO member states. The dream that SARS had fostered of a unified, apolitical commitment to preventing the next pandemic quickly broke down as governments, and the public health professionals who worked for them, retreated into nationalistic corners (Ferguson 1994). The Mexican government reacted particularly strongly, evacuating its citizens from China and accusing Chinese public health professionals of human rights abuses after Mexicans in many cities, including Tianmai, were quarantined and subjected to medical tests for what some were calling "Mexican flu," without reason to suspect that they were infected (Singer 2009).

Thus the efforts that my informants thought would solidify their place in the global health common instead seemed to them to be jeopardizing it. Their bureaucracy had been built for this purpose, people had been trained, money had been invested, infrastructure had been built, and over and over again they had been warned that they were responsible for taming the next pandemic. But now that they were doing exactly what they thought they were supposed to be doing, they were being criticized rather than praised. Worst of all, the international community that they had tried so hard to join, and with which they had worked so hard to build relationships, was shunning them for governing the wrong population in service of the wrong common. Meanwhile the U.S. CDC, which they so admired as the model for their own institution and which represented for them the epitome of scientific modernity, seemed now to be standing by and doing nothing, allowing the disease to invade China.

To many of those working so hard to institute Tianmai's swine flu measures, this felt like a betrayal from the very people who were supposed to be setting an example for professionalized trust. True professionals, my interlocutors had thought, trusted even those in the professional common whom they did not know because true professionals could be counted on to fulfill their end of a bargain, regardless of interpersonal dynamics or personal impact. Their foreign partners had violated these principles. "The international community should support us. This is both in accordance with our own laws and with the [WHO's] International Health Regulations. It's the United States they should criticize; they are the ones who did not do anything to stop this," one TM CDC member told me.

One Step Forward, One Step Back

May 6, 2009

We stand at the front desk of the hotel waiting for the ambulance to arrive, the two of us still in our masks and white coats with the Tianmai CDC logo on the breast pocket, the American tightly clutching her purse and a computer bag—the only items she had brought with her for what she had thought would be a day trip to Tianmai. I say to Dr. Han that the foreigner seems quite cooperative, and she says, "Yes; in contrast to many of the people they have to deal with in Tianmai, her *suzhi* is very high." She says she feels sorry for this woman, who has to go to quarantine for a week all alone without any companion and yet cannot even speak Chinese. She says if the positions were switched, and she were in the United States and the Americans wanted to quarantine her for a week simply because she was on the same airplane as someone with a suspected case of flu, she would be terrified. But it's *meiyou banfa* [there's nothing to be done]!

Han gets a call on her cell phone that the ambulance is almost here. She motions at the American, and then the three of us walk outside in silence, holding our hands to our foreheads to shield our eyes from the blinding May sunshine. When the ambulance pulls up we lead the American down the front steps of the hotel to the curb. She hesitates as the back doors of the vehicle open and two men in biohazard suits, soaked through with sweat, reach out their hands to help her onboard. She turns to me and says "I have to go in there?" and I say, "I'm afraid so," and she lets out a little high-pitched laugh as the men take her arms and gently help her into the back. We wave goodbye. The men in the sweaty biohazard suits pull the back doors closed, and the ambulance turns on its siren and drives away.

In describing his experience in a Chinese quarantine in July 2009, Jonathan Metzl drew on the trope of the backyard farm when he wrote in the *Los Angeles Times*, "The Chinese media have reported that travelers placed in quarantine are being held at five-star hotels, but if this is true, then the star system is in need of revision. Imagine a Motel 6 next to a chicken farm in the middle of a field. Then imagine that it had been left abandoned for a year before receiving a quick cleaning and sanitizing and a lot of new security features." Metzl (2009) went on to charge that by putting healthy travelers like himself into quarantine, the Chinese had acted out of xenophobia and fear. He concluded by declaring that his captors had failed to comply with globally accepted professional norms—just the opposite of what my interlocutors told me they thought they were doing. "Chinese health authorities need to wake up to this lesson and develop China's ongoing H1N1 response in concert with, rather than in rejection of, international norms," Metzl wrote.

Tianmai's public health professionals at first vigorously defended themselves against accusations like Metzl's. Repeatedly they insisted to me that their actions were not rejecting international norms but rather were perfectly aligned with them. They cited WHO plans that presented the SARS response as an example of the kind of global action that should be repeated during an influenza outbreak. They cited the fact that no one knew at first how mild the virus would be, that judgments of severity in any case were not part of WHO preparedness plans—a fact that led to later international criticisms that WHO itself had overreacted to what was essentially an ordinary flu (Reuters 2010)—and that WHO had warned that H1N1 could mutate into something more like H5N1 or might even mix with H5N1 in China. They cited the training that the U.S. CDC and others had given them since SARS and the expectation that they felt came along with this training that they should mount an aggressive response against any influenza threat. They cited pandemic preparedness materials from the Ministry of Health that suggested that, by following the quarantine and containment activities, as well as the surveillance, disinfection, and TCM treatment methods used during SARS, similar results might be obtained for flu (PRC Ministry of Health 2006, 2007a, 2007b). Tianmai's media also stated that WHO endorsed quarantine as a "long-established principle in dealing with infectious diseases" and a "means that can be taken under special circumstances" (Xinhua 2009).

What all of this meant to my informants was that they felt that *they* were the ones who were responsibly carrying out their professional roles to govern risky populations in service of a global common—and thus they were the ones who were deserving not of suspicion, but of trust. On the other hand, just as their colleagues at the lower levels in Tianmai could not be trusted to cooperate in implementing disease control measures within Tianmai, this incident revealed for my informants that their foreign colleagues could not in fact be trusted to cooperate in adhering to the very international standards that they had established and promoted. Those who most demanded service to the global common were not willing, it seemed, to do what was necessary to serve it themselves.

My interlocutors' interpretation of the situation was quite different from interpretations in the United States at the time. Public health officials in the United States clearly did not think that the relatively mild H1N1 outbreak qualified as one of the WHO's "special circumstances" worthy of quarantine and thus did not see implementing quarantine or other aggressive restrictions on population movement as part of their responsibilities, professional or otherwise. What is less clear, however, is what virus *would* qualify. This is difficult to surmise from the preparedness materials that the United States was promoting at the time. Though the U.S. influenza preparedness plan acknowledged that a pandemic could begin in North America, the strategies that it laid out almost exclusively started with the premise that it would begin overseas, most likely in Asia, and that containment measures would be implemented overseas with the goal of preventing or slowing the spread of the disease *from* Asia *to* the United States (U.S. Department of Health and Human Services 2005; U.S. Homeland Security Council 2006; MacPhail 2014).

The plan for U.S. federal government response incorporated this assumption into its own phase system: Phase one of pandemic response would be declared when a suspected human outbreak occurred overseas, whereas phase four indicated the arrival of the virus in the United States (U.S. Homeland Security Council 2006). In an interview that was translated from a *Time* magazine article and reprinted in a local Tianmai magazine at the onset of the H1N1 outbreak, U.S. CDC acting Director-General Richard Besser reinforced this position when defending his decision not to implement any border controls for H1N1: "So at the time that the outbreak was first diagnosed, it was already in the U.S. Our pandemic planning . . . had approached or looked at [an outbreak that] would originate off our shores" (Walsh 2009). The assumption on the part of American public health officials was that, in the event of an influenza pandemic, the population that would need to be controlled on behalf of a global common would necessarily be foreign.

Historian Nicholas King's concept of the "emerging diseases worldview" is instructive here (2002). King suggests that the central principle of "global health" in the late twentieth and early twenty-first centuries was the idea that "we" are all affected and all "in it together" and therefore all need to do our part to combat new diseases. This principle, King argues, grew out of a realization in the 1980s and 1990s that "international" and "tropical" diseases could "emerge" by coming to "us" (the developed world), and therefore "we," as citizens of developed countries, had to care about the spread of such diseases among "them" (the developing world). In keeping with this worldview, the Institute of Medicine (IOM) and the U.S. CDC recommended that the U.S. government attempt to "control dangerous diseases at their source"— the assumed "source" being developing countries in Asia and Africa (IOM 1997; U.S. CDC 2001).

The investment that they had made in training and infrastructure in China, my U.S. CDC and WHO contacts acknowledged, was an important part of this effort to control dangerous diseases at their source. International partners and trainees working in origin countries were expected to work in service of a plan prepared in Western countries and intended first and foremost to benefit those countries. According to these plans, though quarantine of local, non-Western populations on behalf of Western countries might well be appropriate, the possibility of the reverse scenario was not seriously entertained.

U.S. CDC and WHO officials in Mainland China and Hong Kong with whom I spoke agreed that large-scale involuntary measures of the sort implemented in China during both the SARS and H1N1 outbreaks would most likely never be implemented in the United States or any other liberal democracy—except, perhaps, as a last resort (see Gostin, Bayer, and Fairchild 2003; Wynia 2007). U.S. preparedness plans, when describing the conditions under which stringent control measures might be taken domestically, indicated that only if the most basic functions of (American) society itself were at risk would one undertake wide-scale coercive restrictions like blanket border quarantines (U.S. Homeland Security Council 2006; U.S. Department of Health and Human Services 2005). Interviews with U.S. CDC employees supported this view. "At the beginning I got messages asking, 'How is this different from U.S. quarantine?' And I said, 'The United States doesn't quarantine,'" one Beijing-based U.S. CDC employee told me. I asked how high the bar would have to be for the United States to do something along the lines of what he had witnessed in China. Would cholera be reason enough? Ebola? "Yeah, I think there would have to be, like, blood coming out of your eyes!" he replied with a laugh.[4]

Behind the certainty with which American public health officials were able to assert that quarantine was not on the table for a Western response to H1N1 lay a number of basic assumptions. One of these was that large-scale quarantine was not characteristic of a modern approach to disease control but rather was a vestige associated with the past. Many scholars and journalists have noted with amazement that SARS apparently was, as David Fidler (2004) put it, stopped "with essentially nineteenth-century public health instruments" (167). Fidler argued that for a public health response to be sustainable, diagnostics, therapies, and vaccines must eventually replace quarantine. U.S. government scientists agreed; in a December 2009 article, U.S. Department of Health and Human Services Assistant Secretary for Preparedness and Response Nicole Lurie argued that, though quarantine might sometimes be necessary and effective, "the ultimate way to protect individual persons and populations from disease is with vaccination, and the rapid development and manufacture of the H1N1 vaccine represents a triumph of modern science" (2572). Quarantine was presented as an outdated practice that might be used only while awaiting the development of superior technology. Although still sometimes useful, it was not emblematic of the sort of scientific modern disease control apparatus that my TM CDC informants thought they were demonstrating.

Another important assumption with which American officials were working was that Americans and Chinese differed greatly in their willingness to accept an intervention like quarantine. After making his quip about Ebola, the U.S. CDC member interviewed in the preceding paragraphs went on to describe a speech that a colleague had given in Beijing during the initial outbreak, in which he reportedly told Chinese colleagues, "You know quarantine is about risks, and risks that society is willing to take—it's an intervention that's partly determined by your cultural values." An ethical guidance issued by WHO in 2007 supported this cultural relativist stance, suggesting that though all measures that restrict liberties must be implemented only when "strictly necessary in a democratic society," latitude in terms of specific approaches "will depend on local circumstances and community values" (WHO 2007).[5] Gostin and colleagues (2003) have also argued along these lines that "coercive strategies reflect conceptions of individual rights, the legitimacy of state intrusions, and the appropriate balance between security and liberty. Measures tolerable in an authoritarian regime would not be tolerated in a liberal democratic state" (3231–3232). They concluded that, as members of an authoritarian society, Chinese people would find it more acceptable to be subject to coercive practices than people of democratic societies.

Here Chinese public health professionals that institute quarantines and other coercive disease control measures are taken to be representatives of a bounded "local" community writ large, equivalent to Chinese "society" and even to the entire nation-state of China. Chinese colleagues became tied to their compatriots by shared Chinese values that were assumed to naturally trump any shared values that might characterize the professional common of which they thought they were a part or the heterogeneity that the concept of "society" might otherwise imply. By leaving to the judgment of Chinese public health officials which measures were acceptable and which were not, WHO, Gostin, and others presented their cultural relativism as a means of empowering a Chinese community to make its own decisions. One problem with this line of reasoning, of course, is that it assumes the existence of a relatively coherent "Chinese community" of 1.3 billion Chinese. Another problem is that the empowerment of Chinese public health professionals to make their own choices was meant only to apply to how they governed *local* or *national* populations. Once they ventured outside the bounds of the local to take measures that restrained or restricted those with different "values," the rules for acceptability began to change.

In the early days of the H1N1 response, my informants insisted that the values to which they were adhering were—or rather should be—the same as the values of the global health common. Though they embraced the characterization of China as also constituting a kind of community with its own set of coherent values, their membership in a Chinese common and the global health common, they told me, was highly compatible. The lack of democracy in China, as well as a collectivist spirit of self-sacrifice, provided the structural environment needed to implement scientifically necessary disease control measures. The synergy between "traditional" Chinese values, strong Chinese governance, and the "common good" goals of public health should position Chinese public health professionals not as outliers or as deviants but as disease control leaders. Tianmai's public health professionals blamed a democratic system and an emphasis on individualism for the inability of the United States to follow China's lead. Democratic governments would have done the same things China was doing if they were able, they told me.

In explaining why he thought the United States did not quarantine, one TM CDC leader said in an interview:

> In this area, when it comes to infectious diseases, I think that China has better administrative means than the United States—stronger and more effective. If the United States wants to do this sort of thing, it's not easy . . . A lot of our measures, maybe Americans say it's human rights. For example, the current quarantines, they'll say, "I'm not going: you're violating my human rights." Our country, in this area, is clear about having sense. It can take forcible measures.

It was not just the leaders who made this argument. A young worker in the infectious disease department said of the quarantine and other harsh measures, "Some people have been complaining to their embassy, not understanding the situation. But really it's because Chinese leaders are actually one step ahead [*qian yi bu*] of other countries." She pointed to the successful quarantines as an example of China's ability to "walk in front" of the international scientific community by garnering widespread popular support for a more thorough and effective management of potentially infectious populations.

Huang Qing and others argued that Chinese public health professionals were able to take forcible measures, not only because of China's lack of democracy but also because of Chinese people's greater sense of responsibility to collective entities, which they essentialized as a traditional Chinese value. Though this collectivist rhetoric appeared in multiple contexts throughout my fieldwork, the difference here was that during the H1N1 outbreak members of the younger generation, in their eagerness to defend the Chinese approach, were articulating this argument just as often and as forcefully as members of the older generation were. For Huang, the same shared Chinese value that she derided in other contexts as holding her back from reaching her professional potential now was a point of pride when applied to the governance of populations during an outbreak. Just a couple of months after ranting that "Chinese people don't make individual values a priority;

Chinese people want to make you obey, listen to authority, not do anything, be loyal, don't rebel," Huang insisted that these very characteristics made Chinese populations—and even public health professionals like herself—more amenable than their American counterparts to necessary disease control efforts:

> Chinese people are very compliant like that. . . . You say, "You need to be quarantined; we need to take your blood," and they listen to you. They won't go complaining about their individual issues or human rights. Americans, though, think this is about my life, this is me, and my life is very precious and has to be protected, I'm worried about this particular life and have rights, whereas Chinese, we think about the collective and about society—we focus on the benefit to that.

As we saw in earlier chapters, however, this stated ability of the government to control, and the willingness of people to be controlled, was belied by the realities of how the populations that public health professionals managed under more "normal" (*zhengchang*) circumstances behaved. My informants' earlier insistence that contemporary Chinese are *not* always willing to comply, and their accounts of Chinese and foreign patients alike resisting quarantine orders or trying to evade border control, suggested that whatever mass compliance they enjoyed as H1N1 first made its appearance was precarious and anything but essential.

Yet for a brief while at the start of the outbreak, even my younger, well-educated informants abandoned their complaints, suspended their own doubts, and held up their authoritarian system as a model of rational efficiency that should be admired by all. They also proudly told stories of how they were able to convince wary and unhappy foreigners of the necessity of submitting to quarantine, once they explained the scientific logic behind their actions and once they wooed them, as they described it, with the finest accommodations Tianmai had to offer.

Director Lan told me in an interview:

> In the early days indeed there were some who didn't really understand our country's measures. Later, after explaining clearly to them, they can understand the Chinese government's tactics. . . . And we offered them a lot of life conveniences; for example, some wanted to get on the Internet; we bought

them a computer, bought them a cell phone. Some wanted certain products, didn't have clothes; we offered them some, bought them. All food was free. Living conditions were very good; the environment was good. . . . The only thing they didn't have was the freedom to come and go. Everything else could be satisfied.

From my brief experiences working with my CDC colleagues to implement quarantines, I found that these efforts seemed to be relatively effective. The American woman whom I sent to quarantine, although certainly unhappy about going, was cooperative and generally understanding of her hosts' views that this was necessary. And although a few of my interlocutors in both Tianmai and Guangzhou quietly admitted that some foreigners had fought with them or had even run away, forcing the CDC to call the police to help capture them, as one member of the Guangzhou CDC put it, "like criminals," the vast majority of foreign quarantined contacts and patients allowed themselves to be labeled as part of a potentially dangerous population and quietly submitted to their fate. In contrast to the outcry from their governments and their media, for the most part foreign travelers to China accepted the fact that they were now the ones who needed to be governed on behalf of the common good.

Tianmai's successes with placating foreign quarantine patients, however, also reveals the fundamental improbability of replicating Tianmai's model elsewhere. The city's extremely well-funded public health professionals were able to buy the compliance of displeased patients with cell phones, computers, expensive food—anything they wanted. They often explicitly argued that their ability to do so provided evidence that Tianmai had become fully modern and developed. But in almost any other context in China—or anywhere else in the world, for that matter—such a generous compensation program would have been inconceivable.

Furthermore, however rational and generous they felt they were being, public health professionals generally failed to convince one group of people to submit to quarantine: themselves. Xu Dan, for example, admitted to lying about her contact with sick patients and to sometimes taking drugs to mask mild respiratory symptoms when *she* crossed the border between Mainland China and Hong Kong, because she did not want to get caught in her own dragnet. Fu Qiang, an informant in his midtwenties who fell ill with what he insisted was "just a cold" (*ganmao*) while working at the swine flu hospital, admitted to breaking his home quarantine to go shopping because he "felt bored." Several other informants told similar stories. The resistance that Fu and several of his colleagues exhibited when they were asked to comply with quarantine orders themselves revealed the extent to which Tianmai's public health professionals still tended to think of themselves as fundamentally outside the "population." The Communist discourse of self-sacrifice remained important, but sacrifice was defined as the sacrifices that *others* had the responsibility to make: When it came to TM CDC members' own lives, they often were even less willing to sacrifice than their foreign charges were.

The Backlash

May 5, 2009

It is 9:00 p.m., and Huang Qing and I are in the eerily quiet H1N1 isolation ward of the main infectious disease hospital in Tianmai. We are here to meet the latest suspected H1N1 case, a foreign traveler whom the city Quarantine Bureau has brought in from the Hong Kong border. Following Huang's instructions and what I can remember of the emergency training we all attended two months previously, I climb into my protective gear: first the biohazard suit, zipped up, then the N95 mask, surgical hat, and shoe coverings. It is hot, and I instantly begin sweating.

The patient, perhaps sixteen years old, has gently browned skin and a mess of dark curly hair and is lying on a hospital bed, talking animatedly into his cell phone while nurses in biohazard suits take his blood pressure. The nurses report that he does not actually have a fever—his temperature is only 36.9 degrees. "I've been trying to tell them; it's just a headache!" the boy tells me as he puts down the phone. He says he attends a school in Hong Kong and that he had gone on holiday to France—recently designated an outbreak zone—but had returned a full two weeks earlier. He does not feel sick, he says.

Huang, speaking in English, says, "Well, you might have to stay here a little while anyway." He asks how long. A few hours, or maybe a few days, she replies. "A few days? I really don't want to stay here a few days!" Huang replies by paraphrasing the quarantine notice I had helped her to translate the day before, explaining that, for the good of his own health and the health of others and according to international law and the law of the People's Republic of China, he might need to stay for "a while." He becomes quiet, turns to me, and tells me that he is afraid. The nurse is trying to shoo us away so that she can take nasal samples. I don't know what to say, so I just pat him on the hand, tell him not to worry, and we rush out the door. "He obviously doesn't have the virus," Huang says with a sigh, and she rips off her protective gear and throws it in the trash.

July 3, 2009

Lili gets off the phone, exasperated. She says it's all the same—all I can tell them is three things: This flu has symptoms that are the same as a regular flu, go to the doctor, and be sure to do proper disinfection. You see this really is work that should be given to clinical physicians—it should not be the TM CDC's responsibility at all, she tells me. "Our slogan is 'safeguard your health.' It's not 'diagnose your disease.' We do prevention; we serve the group; we don't serve individuals. For that they should go to a hospital, and the hospital should be doing it—it's clinical work!" She groans in frustration. "I still can't bring myself to be polite! Because I just feel so annoyed all the time!"

Although TM CDC leaders continued to insist throughout the summer of 2009 that strict quarantine measures were scientifically necessary, support among ordinary TM CDC employees for enforcing these measures began to falter almost as soon as the virus reached Tianmai in late May. As the pandemic response dragged on, as the United States stopped reporting cases, and as Hong Kong stopped tracking and quarantining contacts, the younger members of the TM CDC began distancing themselves from the rhetoric that their leaders were espousing and that they had at first supported.

Without time to conduct the usual *guanxi* exercises that normally accompanied a major campaign of this sort, the CDC workers in charge of the flu response were relying on local leader pronouncements alone to try to push through the necessary measures. Dismissing *guanxi* requirements as irrelevant in this case, Director Lan insisted that China's "responsibility system" (*wenze zhi*) would assure that something as important as H1N1 prevention would not be ignored by the lower levels—because anyone who did not do his or her part would immediately be fired by upper-level BOH leaders. *Guanxi* rituals, Lan and other leaders insisted, did not play a role in this kind of high-profile emergency situation because the reforms described in Chapter Two had been successful. To the extent that some of the reforms remained incomplete, the benefits of authoritarian rule would take over, Lan implied. Given the very high priority that leaders at all levels had assigned to H1N1 control, lower-level leaders and *danwei* members would follow rules out of fear if not out of professional devotion.

The failure to use *guanxi* to smooth over relations between institutions, however, became increasingly problematic as the summer wore on. Suspicions that those working in the hospitals and clinics were not reporting correct numbers or were dragging their feet in carrying out containment tasks steadily mounted. The most frustration was directed toward parallel municipal institutions responsible for other aspects of the flu response. The relationship between the TM CDC and the Tianmai Quarantine Inspection and Control Bureau, the latter of which was in charge of policing the borders and sending potential flu cases to Tianmai's infectious disease hospital, was particularly tense. Because no one wanted to be responsible for letting the first flu case into Tianmai, everyone was trying to deflect that responsibility onto someone else. Thus, the Inspection and Quarantine Bureau sent even those travelers who did not meet any of the criteria of a suspected flu patient but whom they judged to "look a little sick" to the hospital, angering the CDC personnel who were required to investigate every case.

Foreign patients' complaints and demands also began to wear on my informants' patience and on their confidence that they—or rather their superiors—held the moral high ground. Yet their leaders, ever more eager to show the breadth and depth of the TM CDC's capabilities and to make sure they were not blamed for letting the virus into China, announced almost daily additions to the set of tasks allocated to the increasingly unenthusiastic corps of young people. The twenty-four-hour telephone and laboratory shifts carried on long after the sense of urgency faded. Dashes to the hospital faded into weeks living in hospital dormitories. The weekend overtime to call and check up on every traveler who had entered Tianmai from Hong Kong carried on even as Hong Kong stopped isolating those who felt sick.

The burden of all of these activities fell on the newest, youngest, and most well-educated members of the CDC, who had trained in the shadow of SARS, organized outbreak simulation exercises, attended emergency management trainings, and chased after false alarm after false alarm of avian flu, only to suddenly wonder what the point of it all was. They began to feel silly, frustrated, and finally bitter. They wondered why they were spending so much time on H1N1 while they were more or less ignoring more prevalent and possibly more dangerous diseases that circulated in Tianmai every summer—such as hand, foot, and mouth disease, which had been on the rise for years. They wondered when they would be able to return to their individual research projects. As more and more of their international colleagues abandoned any measures that approached theirs, they no longer felt that Tianmai was "walking ahead" of the rest of the world. They no longer felt like heroes, either. As Fu Qiang, who had once clamored to be assigned to the H1N1 response team, told me over dinner one night in early July, "The leaders are the only ones who get to be heroes. We only get to be cannon fodder [*Zhiyou lingdao cai keyi dang yingxiong. Women zhi neng dang paotui*]."

These disgruntled public health professionals knew exactly whom to blame. The responsibility system of which Lan spoke did seem to temporarily scare public health leaders at all levels into doing what they had been assigned to do. And the authoritarian display of power that their international colleagues had admired them for was more efficient than ever. The problem, these informants told me, was that this display of responsibility reflected neither *renqing* nor professionalism. Their appeals for cooperation without *guanxi* had produced cooperation without rationality, professionalized trust had retreated to state-enforced fear, and straightforward pandering had replaced careful negotiations along the hierarchy.

The result was no more truthful or scientific than what they had started with and yet was also devoid of the human feelings that otherwise made authoritarian rule more fragmented and less efficient, perhaps, but also more tolerable for many. Hierarchically organized *guanxi* responsibilities remained, but the feelings that made them seem meaningful were, for the moment at least, diminished. According to Dr. Yang, an infectious disease specialist at a district-level CDC, "What they're doing, it's not necessarily what they *feel* . . . Because everything you do you're listening to orders; if the leaders say it's right, you say it's right, and if the leaders say it's wrong, what do you do? Right. You don't maintain the truth like this." Because each level of leadership was in turn only responsible to the leader directly above, the main goal of even the most well-educated, rationally minded leaders was not to find the "truth" but to please the leader on the next rung on the hierarchy. Despite the name "responsibility system," during the outbreak this was accomplished primarily through authoritarian fiat rather than through the exercise of agentive responsibility or professional accountability.

The political nature of public health practice had always lurked beneath the surface of Tianmai's public health projects. As employees who depended on the local government for their salary and benefits, my informants were deeply attuned to the fact that, ultimately, they were all part of the long arm of the state. Yet with H1N1, the practice of public health seemed to many to degenerate into a crudely political game in which fledgling attempts at science and professionalism were quickly discarded. Said Dr. Ying:

> The problem is that they are *bugou kexue* [not scientific enough]. For example, with something like H1N1, beforehand you do a lot of research, study what is being done abroad, study the system, come up with a plan. But when something actually happens, they [local colleagues] forget the plan altogether; no one actually follows the plan, instead they do whatever the leader says, which has nothing to do with the plan. And then, when it's over, no one looks at what was done and tries to evaluate the response. If the leaders are satisfied, that's good enough.

These frustrations bubbled to the surface as soon as the first cases of H1N1 inside Tianmai were confirmed in late May. Two Chinese-American tourists headed from Hong Kong to visit relatives in another Pearl River Delta city were stopped at the border after allegedly trying to cover up low-grade fevers with ibuprofen and were brought to the receiving hospital in Tianmai. Fu Qiang, who had been up all night dealing with the situation, told me that the patients "didn't cooperate at all, they were really angry . . . We gave the girl a computer that one of the nurses found in the hospital and bought her a cell phone. We had to! Whatever they wanted basically we tried to give them, anything to make them cooperate and calm down."

The night of the tourists' arrival, I was out of town. Lili sent me a text message telling me that the first case in Tianmai had finally been confirmed, and tensions had immediately boiled over: "Haha, the atmosphere here is really nervous and excited because a case [of H1N1] has finally happened. When the two cases arrived, the leaders got nervous and immediately started yelling at people; it's sort of funny," she wrote.

By the time I returned two days later, however, the atmosphere no longer seemed "funny." Xiao Chen was complaining about the overtime that an enterprising young "emergency management team" leader was putting her through, "all to make himself look good." Lili complained about having to stay up all night answering a hotline that she thought should rightfully have been the domain of clinical medicine: "People keep calling and saying they have a sore throat or a cough and did they have H1N1. I can't tell them anything except to see a doctor—you know we're not the emergency rescue team [*jijiu*]!" Department heads whose employees had all been taken away to work on the flu response, or whose staff had been diverted from more prevalent diseases to focus on tracking flu cases, began to lose patience. One department head told me:

> Everyone's been taken away to do this swine flu thing—we have people in the lab, sleeping here twenty-four hours a day, so obviously it is affecting our work . . . [but] all of the cases here have been so mild that they don't even notice that they're sick! So we're trying to catch people who feel fine and then tell them they're sick and make a big fuss. Meanwhile, they are already better by the time they're even treated! This virus is no SARS.

Abandoning their earlier nationalistic rhetoric and looking to reclaim a place in the global health common, my younger informants increasingly charged their leaders with failing to follow international standards after all. If the U.S. CDC was not responding to H1N1 in the way that the TM CDC was, then it must have its reasons, they told me—it was, after all, the epitome of scientific modernity and the model for their own institution. Because of their leaders' failure to be scientific enough—and because of their overzealous embrace of a Chinese cultural identity and the values of authoritarian control that this identity was supposed to imply—they had lost face with the global health common. In fulfilling the stereotype of Chinese government officials as nothing but arms of a police state, they had lost the chance to prove that government public health workers could be scientists too.

"The leaders need to change their strategy," Dr. Qiu, an epidemiologist in his midthirties, complained. "You can see they're not paying attention [to H1N1 in the United States]. In China, every day they have a count, say there are so many in the United States and so many in China. But in the U.S. papers I look at online, they have nothing!" When I asked Qiu how such a change might occur, he shook his head, repeating the refrain I had heard all year: "There's nothing we can do about it; it's all determined by the leaders." Fu Qiang told me that the problem was not so much with the leaders themselves as with what he called the "irrational system" in which they all operated:

The defect with our system is that there's no way to change something once it's no longer useful. It's fine if you need to adjust a policy, there's nothing wrong with it—back then maybe it made sense [to do all these things we are still doing]. But now it doesn't, but no one's going to stop, because there's no way for anyone to stop; everyone just listens to the leaders, and the leaders are worried only about losing face. There's no process for anyone to adjust; it's completely irrational. That's why it's better in the United States to at least have a process; if something no longer makes sense, you change it, you follow scientific research, get experts to research this problem and decide what is the rational [*heli*] way of proceeding, and then change the policy. . . . [here] they can only start something, but they can't ever stop it. Because they don't know how to stop—no one is willing to take responsibility for doing that.

According to Fu, in an effort to avoid being on the wrong end of the "responsibility system," everyone tried to avoid taking on any responsibility at all. In this way, changes—even changes that everyone knew should be made in the interest of a better epidemiological, economic, and political outcome—could never be made. In short, Tianmai's public health leaders had failed to become professionals.

One day in July I sat down with Dr. Liang, who was in charge of flu response at the same district CDC where Dr. Ying worked. Until May he had been the head of the HIV department, but when the flu hit and Ying happened to be away in Gansu province (near Sichuan) helping with earthquake relief, Liang found himself suddenly at the helm of the flu response. His desk was still tucked away in a small dark room that he shared with his one young assistant, and his cubicle was piled high with papers. He had the appearance of one who had neither slept nor bathed in days. Young women scurried back and forth to his cubicle, leaving reports and asking for further directions. I recognized one of the women from one of my stints in the infectious disease hospital, and we exchanged friendly nods before she disappeared with a briefcase-sized rolling suitcase, headed back to the hospital for another two weeks of twenty-four-hour duty.

Dr. Liang had not slept the previous two nights, he said, because he was busy tracking down the contacts of a Chinese-British businessman who had crossed over the border from Hong Kong to attend a meeting and banquet with dozens of other people. The man had gone to the banquet even though, Liang said, he had already begun experiencing flu symptoms. Some of the man's contacts were not willing to go into quarantine, and Dr. Liang had had to call the police to "catch" (*zhua*) them and "persuade" (*shuifu*) them to go.

Dr. Liang peered wistfully at me as I expressed sympathy for his plight. "The United States isn't doing these things, is it?" he asked. I shook my head. "And I heard even Hong Kong stopped chasing people?" When I nodded, he launched into the same recitation of the reasons for Tianmai's continued strong response that so many of his colleagues had given me. There were too many people in China, and especially in Tianmai the "population was too crowded." China's facilities were not as good as those in the United States. They did not have as many resources, and so prevention was their only hope. Then he stopped, seeming embarrassed, and sighed. "Actually, it's not so much these things; it's just that here all the decisions flow from the upper levels down to the lower levels. The leaders prioritize this, so there's nothing to be done about it; we also have to prioritize it."

Dr. Liang followed up with the familiar statement, *meiyou banfa, dou shi lingdao anpai de* (there's nothing we can do about it, it's all arranged by the leaders). And yet it was clear that, despite the insistence of so many at the city and district levels that nothing could be done, something could, and was, being done at the lowest levels of the hierarchy. Community-level public health and medical system workers and leaders alike were not complying with the city leaders' mandates. They increasingly did not prioritize H1N1 beyond keeping up basic appearances, they avoided reporting cases, they sent their suspected cases back to the TM CDC rather than dealing with them themselves, and they sometimes even failed to organize required trainings or send patients for required tests. They had taken it upon themselves to do exactly what Dr. Liang and Fu Qiang said could not be done: to decide that the mandated response did not make sense or was otherwise unappealing to them and that they were not going to implement it.

Rather than showing solidarity with these colleagues and interpreting their moves as brave efforts to buck irrational demands, however, public health professionals at the city and district levels mostly just continued to express the same contempt they had expressed during previous refusals of the lower levels to cooperate. They insisted that the lower levels' failure to comply was born not of good professional judgment or pioneering individuality but of a type of selfishness that was distinct from their own efforts at professional self-development. From their perspective, although their focus on developing themselves through research and training strengthened the professional project and contributed to the building of collegial trust, the lower levels' efforts to prioritize their own needs weakened that project, promoted corruption, and produced lies. Feeding these allegations was the fact that many of the leaders at the lower levels were older bureaucrats and "technicians" who were not as highly educated as my informants at the city and district levels and not as committed to the same kind of professional project.

Embracing foreign critiques of the Chinese government that painted it as all powerful, Tianmai's public health professionals also placed the blame for their own feelings of inadequacy as scientists on a supposedly tyrannical system in which they were helpless victims. Western observers were right: China was an authoritarian system, and authoritarian values made professionalization impossible, they told me. Dr. Ying told me, "Our Party, their power is great, to the point that it doesn't resemble a party, it resembles a religion . . . if the leader wants him to do something, he has to do it . . . even if you think this is irrational, you still have to do it."

Insisting on their powerlessness in this situation, and appealing to Chinese values of respect for hierarchical leadership, both the older and younger generations of public health professionals at the TM CDC told me that the only way to end the cycle of bad behavior at the local level was for the nation's highest leaders to change their directives. As the virus slowly made inroads all over China in the summer of 2009, it increasingly appeared that this would in fact happen.

When the national CDC began to abandon quarantine as a strategy and to loosen its surveillance requirements, however—acknowledging by July that the disease had spread too far to be stopped—Tianmai's leaders continued to require detailed reporting and quarantining of contacts. An interlocutor who worked for the central China CDC told me: "We keep telling [local CDCs] that they don't need to chase every single contact anymore. They don't need to test every single person who has any symptoms, either. Actually, they never needed to do that. So we need to explain this to them, but, at the local level, it's hard for them to understand; they are worried about face." Eventually, however, the TM CDC leaders seemed to acknowledge that their efforts to show just how modern and scientific their pandemic response system was, and to exhibit just how much they were "walking ahead" of everyone else, somehow ended up showing just the opposite. Late in the summer of 2009, the TM CDC leaders quietly closed Tianmai's quarantine facility, the hospital teams were sent home, and the twenty-four-hour hotline was shut off. The containment effort was over.

Conclusion: H1N1 and the Common Good

Tianmai's public health professionals insisted that, for such a politically important campaign, they could not disobey their leaders and slow down their H1N1 containment efforts. But this does not explain why national and local leaders themselves took such a strong stance in the first place. Why did the leaders persist for so long in taking actions that other members of the global health common almost unanimously agreed, by one or two months into the pandemic, were unnecessary, unproductive, even wrong? Why, even after national level leaders ended most containment efforts, did local leaders in Tianmai continue to compel their highly educated young new hires, to whom they had devoted so much funding and so much cultivation, to do something that those young people found so antiscientific and so contrary to their professional project? How, after all the years of working to gain the respect of the global health common, did they still manage to become yet again, at least for a couple of months, global pariahs?

One obvious explanation is that for all the charges of irrationality, the initial TM CDC response was actually a quite rational consequence of building a public health system that was organized explicitly around emergency response and especially around emergency response to flulike outbreaks. At the beginning of the H1N1 response, TM CDC leaders and members alike felt that they had to take the most aggressive measures possible against H1N1: This was what they thought was demanded by the principles of preparedness in which they had trained and by their roles as members of a global health common. That the Director-General of WHO, Margaret Chan—formerly the Director of Health of Hong Kong—came to power based on her aggressive actions to contain SARS in Hong Kong in 2003 only reinforced the perceived importance of this approach. The conflict between two enduring lessons that my informants took away from SARS—that they should act with scientifically informed professionalism on the one hand and that they should unleash their authoritarian mobilization capabilities on the other—left them feeling betrayed by both their leaders and the international community.

There was another side to this, however. In November and December 2009, as H1N1 became commoner than the common cold throughout the United States, the same Western media outlets that had declared China's measures to be inappropriate began to suggest that perhaps they had been wrong. In a November 11, 2009, *New York Times* article entitled, "China's Tough Flu Measures Appear to Be Effective," journalist Edward Wong noted that, apparently as a result of the strict quarantine measures they took, China's total case count was dwarfed by that in the United States. Wong went on to quote WHO Beijing office director Michael O'Leary as asserting, "I think there were a variety of measures put in place by different countries, and it's difficult to say what worked best and what didn't, but China's has worked very well." Aggressive containment measures, it seemed, could perhaps be "rational" after all. In a more guarded assessment Lurie (2009) argued, "Many observers think that China's isolation and quarantine policy, like the school closures in the United States, was disruptive. Unfortunately, we do not yet have adequate data to help us understand whether any of these measures worked, nor do we have a good understanding of the levels of individual or social disruption that are acceptable to different people, communities, and countries" (2).

Lurie presented this as a simple case of different strokes for different folks. But the divergence of global, national, and local responses to the H1N1 pandemic of 2009 left a far more significant imprint on Chinese public health than this assessment would imply. The unwillingness of the United States to support or participate in the very response that Tianmai's public health professionals thought that country's premier public health institutions had trained them for represented for my informants not only a betrayal of professionalized trust but also a betrayal of the Tianmai dream. Working at the TM CDC, it appeared, did not make them into cosmopolitan, transnational scientists—it just made them into ordinary powerless Chinese bureaucrats, cogs in an authoritarian wheel who were special only in that they were more likely than others to get blamed for the next scary disease that came along. Their foreign colleagues could not be trusted any more than their Chinese colleagues could. Their leaders were not the rational, committed, respectable scientists that they had painted themselves to be when the new recruits were invited to join the TM CDC team. Their idealized dream community in shambles, their transnational personhood threatened, Tianmai's public health professionals dissolved back into a generalized Chinese population, no different in the eyes of the foreign Other than the reviled floating population and suddenly powerless in the face of an all-powerful government.

This brings us back to the problem of the common good. The response to the H1N1 pandemic, the first flu pandemic since 1968, was supposed to be a model for an effective post-SARS global disease control response. This was to be global health at its best: professional scientists, committed to the ethical demands of ensuring the very survival of humanity, working together to govern populations around the world in a coordinated and evenhanded global response. But this dream of the global health scientist serving the global common almost immediately broke down once the origins of H1N1 were identified and the response got underway. Subtle and not-so-subtle accusations of blame or wrongdoing bounced back and forth among those who had sworn to collaborate. The demands of national and local governance ran up against the demands of global service, and the demands of national and local service ran up against the demands of global governance. H1N1 reinforced the identity of China as a population doomed to serve a global common that would only continue to exclude it.

Meanwhile, because of the global scale of the response and the sheer size of the populations considered at risk for the new disease, national "communities" that were assumed to have fixed personalities and shared values became the key players in this game. Global health relies on national and local public health systems to carry out its agreed-upon tasks—not even WHO has the authority to direct the world's disease control professionals to carry out any particular set of measures. Allowances thus had to be made for "local" (that is, non-Western) ways of doing things. The supposed divergence in shared values across national "communities" then transformed a paradigmatic global health response into a series of fragmented public health responses, as the global health common dissolved into an acrimonious collection of representatives of local (or national) interests, organized along familiar lines of geopolitical power. Those who did things in their local ways could feel free to continue to do so only in the interest of controlling their own populations.

The control and governance of populations also ran into the problem of the individual subject. Wong implied in his *New York Times* article that the scientific basis for border quarantines was in debate long after the pandemic had abated. But whether China's actions were scientifically sound in terms of statistically reducing or preventing H1N1 cases in the population at hand was hardly relevant in the end. What kept Tianmai's public health professionals up at night for three months—literally and figuratively—was the question of whether the people who made up those populations were willing to cooperate in this statistical prevention game. In the end, individual agency proved to be critical to the governance of populations after all. Public health professionals could not govern the population without also caring for individuals. And they could not serve the common without allowing for its internal diversity—those aspects of the common that were not, in fact, in common with each other. Without a cohesive global common or a governable population, Tianmai's public health professionals were left wondering once again whom they were serving, and whom they were governing.

Conclusion

Caring for the Population

The question of to whom and for what professionals are or should be responsible has occupied social scientists for a long time. Durkheim (1992) saw the professions as a moral light, a critical foil to the utilitarian demands of the market and the power of the state. Much of this moral light emanated from the responsibilities that professionals developed to *each other*: "It is this discipline that curbs him, that marks the boundaries, that tells him what his relations with his associates should be," Durkheim wrote (14). The physician-anthropologist Paul Farmer (2003) insists that health professionals above all else should be responsible not so much to each other but rather to the poorest of the poor and the most desperate of the sick. Both views of professional responsibility diverge from more cynical views that deny any moral project at all (Illich 1975; Larson 1977; Starr 1982). Larson (1977), for example, suggested that professionalization is about building a "professional project" of social mobility, market control, and prestige—that is, about being responsible only to the self.

As we have seen in the preceding chapters, these models for professionalism are not mutually exclusive. Public health professionals in Tianmai were simultaneously pursuing a professional project and a moral project. On the one hand, they wanted to build careers, achieve social mobility, and become globally reputable scientists. On the other hand, they also wanted to remake professional ethics and rethink their moral commitments. The ultimate outcome of my interlocutors' professional and moral projects, however, bore little resemblance to Farmer's entreaty to serve the poor. Instead, it coalesced around the protection of a city and a way of life that had come to represent China's modernist cosmopolitan ideal, from the threat of a poor migrant majority that instantiated its continued backwardness. Professional responsibility became bifurcated, with service to colleagues, peers, and mentors on one side and the governance of everyone else on the other.

Throughout this book I have suggested that many of the ethical challenges that this bifurcation of service and governance produced are not unique to China. Debates surrounding rights that should or should not be afforded to unauthorized immigrants, for example, rage on in the United States (De Genova 2002; Willen 2007; Castanada 2010), as do debates about the treatment of research populations (Brandt 1978; Rothman 2000; Petryna 2009), concerns about the fabrication of data in research (Carey 2015; Foster 2015), and arguments over how to balance civil liberties and disease control priorities (Weiser and Goodman 2014; Rothstein 2015).

Within China, these challenges are reflected in many of the country's other emerging professions as well, including law, business, and medicine. In discussing the modern development of the professions more generally in China, Alford and Winston (2011) suggest that "professionalization may happen because it is driven, willy-nilly, by certain elite groups that have adopted a global orientation and that interact on a regular basis with their counterparts in Western countries. These groups may fail to serve large segments of the Chinese population, who are in as much need of professional services as anyone else but are not able to command them" (18). This observation, which *Infectious Change* largely supports, leads them, as it does me, to a simple question: "Can Chinese professionals sustain a commitment to public service and not just occupy an occupational niche?" (18). Or, in the case of public health in Tianmai after SARS, can Tianmai's public health professionals commit themselves to serving the populations they are governing?

The events that I trace in this book point to at least two steps that Tianmai's public health professionals could take to accomplish this goal, if they so chose: First, they could work to eliminate the distinction between service and governance—and thus between the "common" and the "population"; second, they could expand the boundaries of public health to include a commitment to the individuals who make up the aggregate "client" that public health professionals serve.

These should not be impossible tasks. The interests of the individual have taken on great importance in the years since Mao's death. In fact, China scholars have heralded the "rise of individualism" as one of the most important trends of the late reform period in China (cf. Ong and Zhang 2008; Yan 2009). And, as we have seen throughout this book, face-to-face *guanxi* interactions between two individuals continue to be critical to how public health projects are accomplished in China (and indeed, to some extent, anywhere). The individual has never been far from the Chinese public health professional's mind.

The history of public health in both China and the "West" also includes plenty of precedents for service to vulnerable populations. In both settings, modern public health had its roots in a moral commitment to improving the conditions in which poor and disadvantaged populations live. Historians of public health in the United States and Europe have charted how efforts to control disease had, by the nineteenth century, become entangled with a commitment to improve the lot of the poor (Rosenberg 1987; Rosen 1993; Tomes 1998). In China, the barefoot doctor movement and the Patriotic Health Campaigns were both organized around serving the country's poorest citizens.

With this history in mind, some public health reformers in China have attempted to revive the spirit of "serve the people" through appeals to an extant Communist ideology. In a speech at a conference I attended in Tianmai in November 2008, for example, a local professor of public health explicitly called for a return to the Patriotic Health Campaigns as a model for how Chinese public health professionals could control infectious diseases after SARS and "serve the people" at the same time. "That is our tradition," he explained.

A wider commitment among public health professionals to "serve the people" is not likely to be accomplished with appeals to the past, however. Not only did my informants reject nearly everything to do with the period of Mao and his mass campaigns, but the bits and pieces that they did incorporate into their own discourses of self-sacrifice and collective benefit were applied selectively in ways that potentially undermined, rather than facilitated, a goal of serving Tianmai's more vulnerable populations. For the younger members of the TM CDC in particular, self-sacrifice became something that *others* were primarily responsible for doing. Although they might be willing to make significant sacrifices at the height of an acute emergency response, they had little will to do so during the drudgery of a prolonged disease control effort or when faced with the potential of becoming entrapped by their own quarantines. Instead, they expected the same population that already was sacrificing to build their city and drive their economy—the floating population—to accept the mantle of self-sacrifice in the realm of public health as well.

The Western mentors and colleagues with whom Tianmai's public health professionals collaborated and whose behavior they modeled did not set much of an example for how to serve local populations, either. They exhibited even less willingness to sacrifice themselves or their compatriots for the good of vulnerable Chinese populations and offered little evidence, in the Chinese context at least, of the social justice motivations so often associated with global health service. Those from Western countries who were interested in helping the world's poor tended to go to more obviously needy places—sub-Saharan Africa, South Asia, Latin America—rather than to China. The status of China as a global power and the ability of the Chinese state to carefully manage and shield foreign involvement from many of its domestic problems ensured that foreigners involved in public health projects in China were more likely to be engaged in research and surveillance than in humanitarian aid.

Yet models for service did exist, even within the confines of the TM CDC. A small group of public health professionals in one department of the TM CDC, for example, was attempting to promote service to vulnerable populations by drawing on the strengths of Chinese ethical systems already in place: that is, *guanxi* and *renqing*. By engaging more directly with individual suffering on an intersubjective level, nurturing *renqing* with members of the "population," and creatively employing *guanxi* rituals, they directed the moral energy that all of Tianmai's public health professionals possessed in some form toward service to some of what Jean-Luc Nancy (1991) calls the "potential communities" that surrounded them. Haiyan Lee (2014) argues that developing *renqing* with strangers is not foreign to Chinese culture or Confucian ideals. "Human feelings" are strongest for kin and fictive kin, but when strangers are stripped of their baggage as class enemies, backward threats, or belligerent foreigners and are allowed to truly be *seen*, in the Levinasian sense, then they too can be targets of compassion, trust, and love.

Cultivating Guanxi *to Serve the People?*

The most unforgettable ones are the *tongzhi* ["comrade"—slang for gay man]
whom we test and then they turn out positive—they haven't had time to prepare
or think through it; they just got tested on a whim. Some of them reacted as if the
whole sky had fallen down. Maybe some of them had thoughts of suicide. Yester-
day I received [a positive test for one]—it was one we met at a bar last year. When
I told him it was positive, his whole expression stiffened. Then he said, "I really
have an urge to commit suicide." At first, because I'm heterosexual, and rather
young, maybe he didn't really trust me, and some people think in this society,
there's no one to talk to; the pressure is great. But after communicating for some
time, and seeing the age he filled in, I said a few things. I said we have the same
birth year, even the same month. He asked what date, and I said just a few days
after yours. I think this closed the gap between us a little.

—XIAO HU, TIANMAI CDC HIV/AIDS WORKER

I talk to them, just *suibian liaoliao* [casually chat], try to ease their *xinli yali* [bur-
dens of the heart] a little. A lot of people are really grateful that we have this sort
of attitude. But often we fail. When I first came, I really welcomed a certain gay
man. We talked a lot about prevention, infection, and so on, and he felt he should
be careful to always use a condom. Six months later he came back and was still
normal, hadn't gotten infected. He was one of the first gay men I met, and because I had just started everything felt new. The second time we also talked for a
long time, and he said he wanted to become a volunteer, do propaganda work, for
AIDS prevention knowledge. I think at the time he thought his future was bright.
But after a year, he came and said he was getting ready to go home; he didn't want
to stay in Tianmai anymore. He wanted to test one more time, and if there was no
problem he'd go home. The results were positive. I felt so defeated. I felt that all
the work I had done before had no meaning. I felt it was very sad [begins to cry].

—XIAO LIU, TIANMAI CDC HIV/AIDS PROJECT COORDINATOR

There was only one department of the ten to which I rotated at the TM CDC where meaningful engagement with, and service to, members of the population to be governed occurred on a daily basis: the Department of HIV/AIDS Prevention and Control.

The international community began pushing the Chinese government to increase efforts to control HIV/AIDS in the late 1990s, and since then organizations, including the U.S. CDC, WHO, and the Gates Foundation, have made slow inroads into China to push their HIV control agendas. But it wasn't until the SARS outbreak in 2003 focused attention on China's failures in infectious disease control that the central Chinese government made a significant push toward openness and action in fighting HIV/AIDS. When then-Premier Wen Jiabao shook hands with an AIDS patient on World AIDS Day in 2003, just months after SARS disappeared from the world, he indicated that AIDS—in keeping with the government's focus on high-profile, globally significant infectious disease problems—would now follow SARS in becoming a "top priority" of the Chinese government.

Local leaders followed suit, competing to show how much *"guan'ai"* (love and care) they could express toward suffering AIDS patients. In Tianmai, for example, the TM CDC director appeared on a television program in 2008 celebrating World AIDS Day and discussed in an interview on the program how it was the job of TM CDC workers to "love and care" for marginalized populations. The program included scenes of Director Lan giving a rousing speech to applause at a crowded gay bar. Around the same time, the TM CDC, TM BOH, and local government leaders staged a four-hour public event celebrating the opening of four methadone clinics for the treatment of heroin addiction in Tianmai as part of the city's HIV/AIDS prevention efforts. Several city leaders made a show of shaking hands with the recovering intravenous drug addicts and publicly expressing their *guan'ai*, while a mother of one of the addicts took the microphone to tearfully thank the benevolent Tianmai leaders for saving her son from drug addiction.[1]

These performances call to mind the Spring Festival performance described in the Introduction, in which heroic TM CDC workers saved earthquake victims from death and destruction in Sichuan and sang of being motivated by "the kind of love that doesn't need words." But although the images of interpersonal salvation that the Spring Festival performance produced did not correspond to the reality of the work that most of Tianmai's public health professionals did, the HIV/AIDS performances publicized on television matched up somewhat better. That is because, in the case of HIV/AIDS, foreign discourses and copious amounts of foreign funding reinforced the "love and care" model for HIV/AIDS control, with foreign collaborators insisting that HIV/AIDS was a biosocial disease that could be effectively controlled only through intensive social intervention (Kleinman et al. 2008).

The result was the development of a parallel discourse, specific to HIV, for what public health in China should do and whom it should serve. Nearly everyone I talked with about HIV both inside and outside the dedicated department at the TM CDC told me that, unlike the other disease threats with which they dealt, "AIDS is not just a disease; it's a social problem." Drawing on international public health messages on the subject, Tianmai's public health professionals told me that this meant that effective HIV prevention and treatment programs had to involve integrated efforts to change individual behaviors, to uncover problematic social structures, and to address social problems such as stigma, as well as political issues, including "human rights."[2] And it had to involve individualized attention to stigmatized Others.

The Tianmai CDC HIV/AIDS department began as a branch of the infectious disease department in 1997, with two dedicated workers who primarily conducted laboratory testing of blood samples. Immediately following SARS, HIV/AIDS broke off into its own department and almost instantly tripled in size, from five to fourteen members. By 2008 it was among the biggest departments at the TM CDC. Most of these members participated at least intermittently in the voluntary counseling and testing service (VCT) housed in an isolated, discreetly marked building on the grounds of the CDC, and even laboratory technicians in the department at least occasionally went "to the field" (*xianchang*) to "*ganshou yixia*" (experience for a moment) testing or outreach in bars, parks, or entertainment centers.

When I arrived in 2008, a team of field workers, epidemiologists, and laboratory technicians staffed the department. Their educational backgrounds ranged from vocational school to doctoral degrees. The leaders placed the HIV/AIDS workers in the department in the same way that they staffed the other departments of the TM CDC—that is, more or less arbitrarily. Those placed in the HIV/AIDS department had *not* arrived at the TM CDC with any greater commitment to the service of local populations than any of the other people I met at the CDC, and they had *not* self-selected or (with the exception of one postdoctoral student) requested placement in the department. They had the same backgrounds and the same range of educational levels as those in other *"jibing kongzhi"* (disease control) departments of the TM CDC (see Chapter Two). Many had worked in other departments before being reassigned, most had little knowledge of HIV before starting, and few had previously met an openly gay man, a sex worker, or an intravenous drug user. "In university we didn't learn much about AIDS, just some theory—but nothing like this," one new young staff member told me, his eyes wide after completing his first intervention at a gay bar.

Yet during the five weeks that I spent with the HIV/AIDS department, many of the people I met exhibited remarkable levels of empathy, sensitivity, and patience for the strangers with whom they were working. Several were quite passionate about helping people who, they acknowledged, were not really treated as persons in the larger society (see Guo 2008; Guo and Kleinman 2011). For the first time during the course of my fieldwork, the majority of the people around me seemed to care deeply about the people who made up the populations they governed—and they cared about them not just as a group or an idea but as socially embedded individuals with their own families, contexts, and subjectivities. As the workers quoted at the beginning of this section demonstrate, in truly "seeing" the Other they were able, and willing, to see these individuals in themselves. They talked over lunch about the sad stories of how particular people they met had contracted HIV. They became rattled when those people fell ill. They admitted to sometimes being kept up at night by what they had seen. And they showed patience, tolerance, and compassion toward the marginalized members of otherwise despised local populations who came through their doors.

Their patience did have limits—most of my informants who worked on HIV/AIDS expected those whom they helped to take responsibility for getting themselves tested, behaving politely, and adhering to treatment if available. In other words, they expected them to exhibit relatively high levels of *suzhi*. They also usually excluded intravenous drug users from their sympathies, regarding this group as devious, violent, and in denial about their own culpability for their infections. They did, however, include other members of marginalized groups, such as gay men and sex workers (Hyde 2007). Largely accepting of discourses pushed by their international partners (and later by the MOH and China CDC) that portrayed homosexuality as natural human variation and HIV infection as resulting from closeted behavior linked to strong societal stigma, HIV/AIDS department members generally did not blame gay men for their own infections. And my informants described prostitution not as a crime but as a tragedy affecting victimized young girls who had been abandoned by their families or lured into the sex trade by devious men.

The great majority of the gay men, sex workers, and drug users who came through the TM CDC doors to be tested were members of the floating population. In fact, the HIV/AIDS department head told me that as of 2008, 93 percent of HIV-positive people living in Tianmai were members of the floating population. Yet, in this context, many of the migrants became sympathetic subjects. "I love this work, love to help people, and a lot of people couldn't help it that they got infected," one young woman who had been working there for about two years told me as she compiled reports in the back room of the counseling center one afternoon. "Of course, you might not say that about a drug user, but the gay men, a lot of people have ideas about them, think they're not normal, but I never felt that way. Maybe because they are young like me, I never had the feeling that they were not normal."

In recognizing a connection between herself and the mostly poor migrant people with whom she worked, my interlocutor also opened herself up to a part of her divided self that so many of her fellow TM CDC members so assiduously avoided—that part that not so long ago was also vulnerable and poor, the part that had not yet quite become the cosmopolitan self that public health professionals were trying so hard to project (see Chapter One). The intersubjective recognition of the Other as a social person not so different from oneself made his disappearance into a threatening population less likely. And the bifurcation of service and governance, so easy to accomplish when dealing with aggregates, was much less likely to happen in a dyadic relationship more akin to that between doctor and patient (see the Introduction).

The HIV/AIDS workers told me that because they took on this burden of responsibility toward individual others, their jobs were more difficult than those of their colleagues in other departments, who dealt only in the abstract. Dr. Ang, who headed the Prevention of Mother-to-Child Transmission program (PMTCT), said that her job was almost—but not quite—as *"xinku"* (difficult, bitter) as her previous job as a clinical doctor in a hospital. As with her clinical job, there were threats of violence—mostly from husbands who found out that their wives were HIV-positive—and there were emotionally draining close interactions with HIV/AIDS sufferers.

Still, Ang acknowledged that her job was less emotionally difficult than those of some of her colleagues in the department who were less able to help the people they were working with. Pregnant women and their partners were guaranteed free drugs regardless of residency status as part of the PMTCT program. But for those not so lucky as to be having a child, lacking a Tianmai *hukou* meant lacking the ability to obtain the free drugs otherwise guaranteed to all those who could not afford to pay under the national Four Frees and One Care HIV/AIDS treatment program (see Chapter One).[3] This greatly diminished the availability of treatment in Tianmai for the majority of the people who sought testing—making it difficult even for those who truly wanted to serve this population to do so. The young people who conducted the tests and informed patients of their positive status were troubled by this fact and were sensitive to the difficulties that HIV-positive people might have in returning to their hometowns to seek out free treatment. One woman said of her experience,

> A lot of people without a *hukou* can't get free treatment. So they wished we would offer that. A lot of people who get this disease, they *hen diulian* [really lost (moral) face], don't have any respect. They would rather die in Tianmai then go home to get treatment. Like I just ran into a patient; his life is already very hard, he lives on 1000 RMB a month, and for one month's medication he has to pay 500 to 600. He said he doesn't have the money to manage it and wishes we could give it to him for free. But we can't do that; all we can do is advise him to go to where his *hukou* is to get the free treatment.

Still, this woman, like the others I interviewed, stopped short of suggesting that HIV drugs should be provided free of charge to everyone regardless of *hukou*, instead citing the official government position that the policy was necessary to uphold order. This is where the boundaries that Tianmai's public health professionals built in other areas of their work remained stubbornly in place. Although it clearly pained at least some of my informants to be unable to help the individuals they had gotten to know, and although they mostly agreed that it made sense from both a disease control efficacy and a clinical treatment standpoint to treat as many Tianmai residents living with HIV as possible, they still appealed to the secular theodicy of the seemingly immutable decisions of government leaders in explaining why they could not help (Herzfeld 1992). "*Meiyou banfa, jiushi zheyang,*" they told me again and again. "There's nothing to be done. This is just how it is."

My informants rather understandably did not see advocating for major policy changes as a viable position to take, given their positions as relatively low-level government employees. Still, as we saw earlier, the system that was supposedly tying my informants' hands was far from the totalitarian dictatorship that they sometimes made it out to be. This is where the wiggle room provided by *guanxi* came in handy. It was within the HIV/AIDS department that I saw the most evidence of people not so much complaining about *guanxi* as trying to use *guanxi* to work around the system they had, with the express goal of helping local populations.

No one worked harder to do this than Chu Zhaoliang, or "Professor Chu," as everyone called him. Chu ran the TM CDC's gay men's outreach program. A slight man in his midforties who exuded the sort of unbounded energy that could exhaust someone half his age, Professor Chu kept a low profile at the TM CDC but commanded fierce devotion from his colleagues in the HIV/AIDS department. Rather than attempting to change the system, Chu took the tools that he found useful from the system and adapted them to achieve his own ends. The most important tool at his disposal was *guanxi.*

For Chu, there were two kinds of *guanxi* rituals that mattered. One was the kind described in Chapter Two, in which Chu participated in banquets and other *yingchou* rituals with other public health professionals to secure cooperation and funding from his leaders and from other *danwei*s for his projects. The other was the kind Chu used to gain support for and from the at-risk gay men to whom he had devoted his career. Chu managed to extend the production of *renqing* out of the boundaries of the professional common and into the community he was trying to serve, in ways that were unusual in the rest of the CDC system.

Chu was an unlikely AIDS activist. He was married, had a son, and was a career bureaucrat, starting at the TM AES twenty years earlier as a sanitation inspector. As I finally learned after several weeks of working with him, he was not actually a professor either, nor was he formally trained in HIV/AIDS or even infectious disease control. Rather, after finishing his bachelor's degree in preventive medicine he worked for years in the environmental sanitation department, testing air and water quality in bars, hotels, and entertainment centers.

While he was conducting these tests during the 1990s, he noted that the venues he was testing for environmental contamination had another, potentially more important health problem brewing: These were the places where sex workers and closeted gay men, both at high risk for HIV/AIDS, came to have sex. Over the years he carefully cultivated his relationships with a large network of bar and other *changsuo* (venue) owners. In 1999 he attended a training session in Hong Kong on how to work with volunteer organizations to provide outreach to those at risk of HIV/AIDS, where, he says, "I learned everything about the model we now use." In 2004, when TM CDC leaders had an opportunity to work with international collaborators to start a *changsuo*-based outreach program for gay men at risk of HIV/AIDS, they tapped Professor Chu to run it.

When I met Chu, his team was busy going out to bars, clubs, and saunas on weekend evenings to collect blood samples and surveys from gay volunteers for an HIV prevalence study funded by a Hong Kong university and several international organizations. Participating in the study gave Chu the opportunity to hand out health education materials and provide a free testing service for those in need, in an environment that was comfortable for them, if foreign and bewildering to Chu's assistants. The research portion of the study was overseen by a PhD student who was working on the project as part of her dissertation research, and she saw to it that informed consent procedures and other bureaucratic rituals, although still imperfect, were completed with somewhat more rigor than those performed in the other contexts I encountered. Perhaps more important, Chu made sure that the focus of each encounter was on education and testing of individual participants, not just on data gathering. Public health interventions and public health research were still being conflated, but the service goals of both were more concretely oriented toward the target population. Chu regularly stepped in to make sure research assistants were protecting anonymity, providing adequate information about how participants could obtain results, and explaining appropriate informational materials.

The model that Chu used to reach his target population and that he said he learned from his training program in Hong Kong involved relying on a close partnership with a local gay men's NGO, one of the few operating at the time in southern China. The charismatic leader of the NGO, a flamboyant computer programmer and one of the only "out" gay AIDS activists in Tianmai at the time, had become one of Chu's best friends, and they joked easily throughout the testing sessions, with the Professor standing in the background overseeing the operation and the gay NGO leader busily rounding up recruits. In exchange for project funding that the CDC funneled into the NGO, NGO members accompanied the CDC workers several nights a week, helping to pull in hundreds of subjects for the project.[4]

Professor Chu had to balance a wide variety of service obligations in these interactions, including service to the foreign members of the transnational scientific common who were providing funding and support for the project, service to the local professional common, service to his NGO partners, and service to the gay population at risk for HIV. But it was the final type of service that by all appearances was driving the project. The *renqing* between Chu and these men was palpable.

Chu encouraged his assistants to talk with the participants in his outreach and research projects, to learn about their lives, and to do whatever they could to make them feel comfortable. He invited the NGO volunteers, many of whom were gay HIV-positive migrants themselves, to eat with TM CDC members before and after the sessions, to chat with them while they waited for participants to sign up, and to befriend his entire research team. This willingness to engage carried over into the voluntary counseling and testing sessions (VCT) that my interlocutors conducted at the TM CDC during regular business hours and resulted in the kinds of intense and moving exchanges documented in the stories recounted by Xiao Hu and Xiao Liu at the start of this section. The result was an overall atmosphere of camaraderie, generosity, and comfort among all three parties: the participants, the NGO members, and the young public health professionals.

The young men and women who made up the HIV/AIDS team drew inspiration from Professor Chu. It was because of Chu, they told me, that they gave up their Friday and Saturday nights to sit in the back room of a gay bar and hand out information on HIV. It was because of Chu's friendships with the gay men that they too were able to think of these men as people, as individual subjects, and even as friends. And it was because of the relationships that they developed that many felt sad and troubled when they could not provide those they served with the drugs that they needed to save their lives.

It is these personalized feelings of moral disquietude that provide a basis for change. Chu made "serve the people" plausible in this small corner of contemporary urban China—not by trying to mobilize the masses or rebuild devotion to the Party but rather by committing to a reintegration of service and governance that rejects the artificial separation between helping a population and helping an individual—and then by building a different kind of professionalism, one relationship at a time.

Chu told me that he took inspiration for the reintegration of the individual into public health from the Mao era—a time that, although full of damaging excess, did allow for the practice of a kind of public health that according to Chu was long-term, patient, and even caring:

> In the 1950s and 60s, before the Cultural Revolution, the AESs did really well. They had a remarkable success in lowering the death rate and stopping infectious disease. The most important aspect of this was *suifang* [follow-up]. They had an excellent system of *suifang*. So, for example, if a child had cholera, they would check on him one week, one month, and even a year afterwards. They followed up. They made sure he was all right. This was extremely effective. All the rates went down. But then with reform and opening, there was a change. We went from preventing and stopping disease to merely "testing" and the sanitation work. The purpose of what people did here changed completely. Then, after SARS, there was another change, and now the CDC is continually changing. But if you really want to see China's successes, you need to go back to the 1950s and 1960s. They really did a good job, because of the follow-up, the care. We don't do that anymore.

In emphasizing follow-up and "care," Chu highlighted the loss of both in the current era of public health. During the Mao period, though campaigns were conducted on the mass level, barefoot doctors provided both preventive services and clinical care, and disease control was integrated with patient care. When public health reemerged as a profession after SARS, disease control and prevention became explicitly separated from patient care. Public health became a problem of the population, not of the individual. Although scholars often portray the reform era as a period of extreme individualism, and contrast it with the collectivism of the Mao period, Chu romanticized the Mao period as a time when such divisions were not necessary and when the prevention and care of both the masses and the individual were seamlessly integrated.

The example of HIV/AIDS work at the TM CDC provides a proof of principle for the possibility of a shift among Tianmai's public health professionals, driven perhaps by inspirational innovators like Professor Chu,

toward an ethic of service, care, and even social justice for vulnerable local populations. Intimately exposing public health professionals to suffering
among marginalized people who in other contexts have been regarded as the
most stigmatized of nonpersons (Guo 2008), and encouraging them to touch
them, converse with them, and learn about them, can make those marginalized people into sympathetic subjects whom one might develop an ethical
obligation to serve. Sparking a sense that something can and should be done
to help those subjects then could be the first steps in reintegrating service
and governance. Spurred to help particular members of a population usually
seen as an infectious threat, a responsibility to serve the population at large
has the potential to develop and spread.

Of course, extending what Chu was doing would not be a trivial task.
Aside from the fact that Chu's charisma was difficult to replicate, my informants almost uniformly told me that HIV/AIDS was a special case requiring special solutions that were not widely applicable to other diseases (see
Nguyen 2010; Benton 2015). International discourses that cast HIV/AIDS
as a biosocial disease requiring both biological and social science-based approaches suggested to my informants—who were trained in a reductionist
tradition and very much bought into the idea that public health problems
were otherwise best approached through biological and statistical methods—
that this disease was the exception rather than the rule. Several informants,
having met other social scientists who studied HIV/AIDS, repeatedly encouraged me to focus my project on HIV/AIDS because "this is a social disease, and you are a social scientist." They seemed puzzled when I suggested
that the same held for all other diseases as well.

In short, Tianmai's public health professionals did not see HIV/AIDS
work as a model for anything other than HIV/AIDS. When after rotating
through the HIV/AIDS department I told members of other departments
of the activities in which I had participated, many were titillated but equally
many were horrified. Several told me that they were glad that they were not
assigned to do the work I described because they felt that, by avoiding such
work, they could avoid the complexities of a "social" disease. And they could
avoid having to interact directly with patients—which, as I have described,
they saw as undesirable and rightfully outside of the realm of their responsibilities. Having observed the emotional and physical exhaustion that their
colleagues in the HIV/AIDS department experienced in interacting with individuals, they chose to stick with populations.

This attitude frustrated those who had hoped that the work they did with HIV/AIDS might lead to a new public health model in China that recognized and dealt with the complex human aspects of *all* diseases. But the powerful apparatus built around SARS provided a compelling alternative to the difficult work that HIV/AIDS required. One Hong Kong scientist who worked on both viruses in collaboration with Mainland scientists explained this problem to me in an interview when discussing the disease control measures that had been enacted to combat H1N1:

> We've spent so much time in the last thirty years showing that quarantine represents only a tiny fraction of the measures you can take to control an infection, and most of the time it's not effective. . . . After going through HIV for all these years, we are trying to understand all the risks in human interaction—this is like a jungle. . . . [but] especially the more I look at the policy makers, they all look so happy now, they've found a tool they can use [quarantine]. In the past twenty to thirty years they may have learned a lot of technical things they can do—infection control, vaccination, sanitation measures, behavioral change—but it's difficult. Not the case for quarantine. It's very easy—you just lock them up.

Expanding Trust

One of the keys to Chu's success, according to both his team and the NGO with which he was partnering, was his ability to gain the *trust* of the people in the at-risk populations he was trying to help. One of the things that would make it difficult to replicate Chu's work was that this trust was closely tied to Chu and his team. Several people involved in Chu's HIV/AIDS work told me that they could not imagine anyone else associated with the local government being invited into such intimate places to do HIV testing. Indeed, Chu told me that the very long hours he worked were necessary because the trust he had won was not transferable to people outside his immediate team. But transferable trust, in the form of what I have been calling professionalized trust and social trust, was exactly what TM CDC's public health professionals were trying, and largely failing, to build after SARS.

Yan Yunxiang (2009) argues that building social trust will require a new type of sociality that must be distinct from the sociality of a system based in personal trust: The dependence on *guanxi* must be replaced by rules and institutions and by the cultivation of a stronger civic commitment among all Chinese citizens. Under this rubric, Chu's approach to trust building was a dead end. But as Shapin (1994) suggests, rules and institutions alone cannot replace the continuing importance—not just in China but everywhere—of personal relationships (see also Gidddens 1990). Many of my older informants saw a danger in attempting to abandon their use of *guanxi*, however corrupt it might seem to some, for the sake of rationality and rules alone. Some of these older informants suggested that trying to do their work without *guanxi* basically was equivalent to trying to do it without any moral guidance at all. They told me they would feel lost in such a world. For whom were they working so hard, and why? *Renqing* ethics made completing public health tasks important because of the obligation that those involved had to their *guanxi* partners. With their responsibilities to the larger population so abstract and so diffuse, the very concrete intersubjective engagements that public health professionals had with their *guanxi* partners and the *renqing* that was produced took on a greater moral force.

Why, then, can't personal trust form the basis for new forms of social and professionalized trust? Mencius argues that "setting up an abstract standard of indiscriminate love without coming to terms with concrete human situations is to ignore the very context in which the ideal is to be actualized" (Tu 1979, 28). As the example of Professor Chu's work suggests, in the context of public health at least, drawing on networks of personal relationships and *renqing* between individual people might be just the way to start building social trust with populations. Until public health professionals and the populations they govern can trust each other on a personal level, they are unlikely to trust strangers in the abstract (Giddens 1990).

Beginning with the familiar *guanxi* rituals associated with sanitation inspections, Chu developed relationships with owners of venues frequented by gay men. Struck by the health implications of the activities that occurred in the businesses they ran and encouraged by his training in Hong Kong and his encounters with global public health discourses on HIV/AIDS risk and prevention, Chu began talking to his *guanxi* partners about his concerns and about possible interventions and began familiarizing himself with the gay community in Tianmai. Eventually Chu expanded his web of interpersonal relationships beyond the usual circle of clients and colleagues to a core group of gay male activists. He did this largely by employing the same methods of banqueting and gift exchange that normally took place between colleagues. By the time he was appointed to run the gay men's outreach program at the TM CDC, Chu had all of the connections he needed to run a successful program.

The benefits of Chu's *guanxi*-building exercises were not only instrumental. Developing personal relationships with members of a marginalized group established these group members as full-fledged subjects and human beings—subjects who shared things with him and in whom he was able see a part of himself. Opening himself up in this way helped his subordinates and colleagues do the same. Establishing these relationships also convinced gay men whom he had not yet met that he was there to help them. In the HIV testing events that I attended, bar owners and NGO activists frequently persuaded the men in the bars and saunas whom my informants were trying to reach to submit to testing by telling them that they knew and trusted Chu and that they could vouch for the his team's good intentions and desire to help. By giving others in Chu's department the opportunity to engage with the men in the same way that he did, and by inspiring them with his infectious enthusiasm, Chu spread this ability to trust to dozens of other people.

This is why my conversations with the members of the HIV/AIDS department were so different from those who rarely had these kinds of interactions. Trust in public health—whether with the public or with other professional colleagues—is not likely to come simply by introducing layers of bureaucratic accountability, as important as accountability may sometimes be. Nor is it likely to come about by cracking down on personal relationships. Chu's work suggested that it is possible that social trust between professionals and populations could begin to arise from real intersubjective engagements with those who are vulnerable and from the desires and moral yearnings of the public health professionals themselves (Giddens 1990). Encouraging these types of engagements will not completely solve the larger crisis of trust that my informants felt had overtaken Chinese society, but it could be an important step forward and would lend greater moral force to the public health professionalization project. As Ignaas Devisch (2013) put it, "The public does not have to coincide with the indifference of a statistic, with being taken up in an anonymous huddle" (105).

Global Health, Global Responsibilities

For all the good work that Chu was doing, his model for interpersonal engagement was not a panacea. The unique challenges of ethically and sensitively engaging with an entire population are inherently different from those associated with clinical work and other occupations that deal only in face-to-face dyadic interactions. Public health professionals around the world often must govern thousands or even millions of people. Even where they do make an effort to engage with and care for individual members of these populations, engaging meaningfully with the suffering or potential suffering of millions of individuals at once is an impossible task. One simply cannot connect with a large aggregate in the same way one can with a particular person, no matter how noble one's intentions, and adding up the interpersonal responsibilities generated by dozens or even hundreds of personal encounters will never produce an equivalent aggregated responsibility.

This disconnect between the interpersonal and the aggregate becomes evident when we examine, for example, which individuals within the marginalized at-risk population the HIV/AIDS team chose to engage (gay men and sex workers) and which they chose not to engage (drug users). The latter group had needs that were just as great as the former, but its members served as less sympathetic characters; in Miriam Ticktin's terms, they were less worthy of compassion (2006). Having been excluded from the building of personal relationships, they also became excluded from my interlocutors' responsibility to the aggregate. As this example makes evident, the whole will never quite equal the sum of its parts, in part because the parts are almost never randomly chosen.

Thus there are clear limits to Chu's strategy of personal, individualized investment and trust acting as a gateway for good public health stewardship. Although the kind of intersubjective service I describe in the preceding paragraphs can perhaps successfully create a *desire* to close the gap between service and governance—and maybe even the beginnings of the trust necessary to accomplish this—effective service requires more than just a willingness to serve. Populations are diverse in their makeup and needs. Even for those who are devoted in principle to serving *all* of those they govern and who have developed a plan for doing so, slippage between those who are served and those who *should* be served all too often occurs. Money does not always go to where it is supposed to, interventions sometimes fail or cause more harm than good, and projects sometimes produce more benefits for funders than for program recipients. Certain more vulnerable members of a targeted population might end up benefiting less from available interventions than those more able—because of education, class, luck, or connections—to navigate the available options (see Whyte et al. 2013). All of this has, in the past and in other contexts, led to serious limitations on who actually ends up being served.

These problems only become magnified at the global level, because of the immense diversity of the populations that global health practitioners often try to serve at once. Service projects developed to aid a poor population in Uganda, for example, might be of little relevance to a poor population in China, and attempting to implement them in both places might inadvertently end up serving neither population (Ferguson 1994; Biehl and Petryna 2013; Farmer et al. 2013; Moran-Thomas 2013). Global organizations also have the challenge of navigating in a multitude of foreign contexts under a multitude of political systems, often without the power of the state behind them. NGOs or other organizations devoted to service in China or in any other country do not have what Hannah Brown (2015) calls "sovereign responsibility." They may form a node of governmentality (Burchell et al. 1991; Kohrman 2004, 2005), but, especially in a place like China, they cannot make use of the formal tools of governance (Zaidi 1999; for a discussion of governmentality and governance in China, see Sigley 2006). Their ability to manage the distribution of services or the measurement of outcomes is dependent on those who do have the mandate to govern—creating a permanent and intractable bifurcation of service and governance, albeit in another form. This bifurcation was particularly pronounced in China, where outside attempts to share governance responsibilities or to provide services not sanctioned through official government channels could be, and often were, much more easily rebuffed by both local and central governments than in poorer and less powerful states more reliant on foreign aid.

Anyone hoping to make a long-lasting difference in global health, therefore—whether by helping the poor avoid what Paul Farmer (1999, 2003) calls "stupid deaths" from malnutrition or treatable infectious diseases, by preventing the next influenza pandemic, by studying cross-cultural cancer risks, or by vaccinating children for measles—must first be willing and able to engage with, and to trust, those local people on the ground who can effectively assess, understand, and ultimately govern the diversity of local populations in need. And those local contacts in turn must find a way to engage with, trust, and be trusted by local populations.

Despite all the obstacles laid out in these pages, of all the myriad global health actors—NGOs, philanthropists, academic researchers, foreign aid organizations, UN agencies, community health workers—local public health professionals still are often in the best position to find an effective way to connect the will to serve with the governance capabilities necessary to effectively and consistently deliver services over a long period of time. They are familiar with their populations, they have a mandate to govern those populations, and, in places like China at least, they have access to the infrastructure needed to serve them as well. As we see with the case of Professor Chu, they also have the ability, if they so desire, to intimately understand at least some of the individual lives that ultimately need to be improved if service to the aggregated population is to be accomplished. In this way, public health professionals like the ones I knew in Tianmai have the potential to become the foundations on which effective and ethical global health cooperation can be built. Understanding the factors that might be holding them back from taking on this role has been an important goal of the present study and, I suggest, is critical to building a more locally sustainable and effective approach to global health initiatives and collaborations.

And yet the onus for effectively and ethically translating global public health projects to local settings cannot be placed on local public health professionals alone. Despite the relatively greater power of the Chinese state and its agents, influence over globally oriented public health programs in China, as we saw in Chapters Three and Four, still often flowed along familiar geopolitical gradients of power. My informants' (mostly Western) foreign partners had a lot more power and influence than they admitted to. As such, those who work with local public health professionals on global health projects in China, or elsewhere, must be careful not to take part in a "division of ethical labor" (Cribb 2009) that attempts to transfer ethical responsibility for the well-being of local people affected by global health interventions to local public health professionals alone.

As the cases of the Great Migrant Study and the H1N1 quarantines make clear, culpability for local ethical breaches all too often has global roots. The exclusion of Tianmai's populations from the common good, their establishment as both biocapital to be utilized and threats to be controlled, the assumption that they will continually sacrifice without necessarily ever benefiting—all of these ethically troubling situations can be traced back, in one way or another, to (usually) well-intentioned global health interventions, trainings, or policies. In partnering with local public health professionals to serve populations around the world, then, global health practitioners must also, necessarily, partner with them to open the black box in which project meets population and look inside with open eyes.

Appendix 1

Tianmai CDC by Department (as of 2009)

Administrative Departments

Main Office
Party Office
Human Resources
Finance Department
Scientific Education Quality Management Department
Public Health Management, Emergency Coordination, and Information
    Department (crossover)
General Facilities Department
Project Office

"Public Hygiene" Departments

Testing and Inspection Services Department
Immunization Management Department (crossover)
Disinfection and Pest Control and Prevention Department

Microbiology Inspection Department (crossover)
Preventive Hygiene Evaluation Department
Environmental Hygiene Department
School Hygiene Department
Nutrition and Food Hygiene Department
Toxicology Laboratory
Genetic Modification Research Laboratory
Chemical Testing Center
Outpatient Clinic

"Disease Control" Departments

Infectious Disease Prevention and Control Department
Epidemiology Department
Public Health Management, Emergency Coordination, and Information Department (crossover)
Immunization Management Department (crossover)
Microbiology Inspection Department and Laboratory (crossover)
Molecular Biology Laboratory and Parasitic Disease Control and Prevention Department (this split up, and Parasitic Disease Control joined the Infectious Disease Department in 2010)
Health Education Department
HIV Research Laboratory
HIV/AIDS Prevention and Control Department

Appendix 2

Glossary of Chinese Terms

aiguo weisheng yundong Patriotic Health Campaign

baijiu Chinese rice liquor

changsuo venue

chengzhongcun village-in-the-city, urban village

chijiao yisheng barefoot doctor

chiku eat bitterness (endure hardship)

chuangshou earning money/for-profit

chuangzaoxing creativity

chuli yiqing deal with or investigate an outbreak situation

danwei work unit

dazhuan vocational college

diu lian/diu mianzi lose face

duguo shu educated, have received an education

fangbao ke hospital disease control department

fangyi epidemic prevention

fangyizhan Anti-Epidemic Station (AES)

fazhan ziji develop oneself

fuyou baojian maternal and child health

fuyou renkou wealthy population

ganqing emotions

gaodu zhongshi to make a top priority

gonggong weisheng public health/public hygiene

gongwuyuan civil servant

gongyi common good, public benefit

guan'ai love and care

guanxi personal relationships that carry reciprocal obligations

heli rational

hukou household registration

huoluan major instability

jiance inspection, detection

jiandu oversight, supervision

jiankang jiaoyu health education

jiankang zheng health license, health certificate

jibing kongzhi disease control

jibing yufang kongzhi zhongxin Center for Disease Control and Prevention (CDC)

jichu yixue laboratory medicine/basic medicine

jiedai keren entertain guests

jingji fazhan economic development

jingshen spirit

jishu renyuan technician, technical worker

jiti collective

jitizhuyi jingshen collectivist spirit

jiu wenhua culture of alcohol, drinking culture

juemi top secret, completely secret

juweihui residents' committee

kai hui to hold a meeting

kan bingren to see patients

keti/keyan scientific research project

kexue science

konghuang panic

kuai-kuai horizontal structure

li ritual

liangxin conscience, remembering and acting on moral obligations

linchuang yixue clinical medicine

lingdao leader, official

liudong renkou floating population

liudong renkou chuzuwu guanli suo floating population rental management bureau

luan chaotic

manxingbing chronic disease

mianzi face (as in "losing face")

nongmingong peasant workers (often indicating migrant workers)

paiwai excluding outsiders, discriminatory

qing ke to treat, invite

quanbu bokuan complete funding (for example, government funding for an institution)

quanguo weisheng zhuanye jishu zige kaoshi National Health Professional Skills Qualification Exam

qunti group, subpopulation

qunzhong the masses

ren humaneness, benevolence

renkou population

renkou wenti population problem

renmin the people

renmin jiankang the people's health

renqing human feelings

renqun crowd, group

renzhen hardworking

richang gongzuo everyday work

shehui society

shequ community (administrative)

shequ weisheng fuwu zhongxin or *shequ jiankang fuwu zhongxin* Community Health Service Center

shi/qu/jiedao city/district/"street" levels of administration

shiye danwei technical work unit

shou or *shuxi* close (as to a person)

suifang follow-up (care)

suzhi (di/gao) quality (of a person) (low/high)

tiao-tiao vertical structure

tijian physical examination

tongzhi "comrade," slang for gay man

wailai renkou "outside population"

wei renmin fuwu "serve the people"

weisheng jiandusuo Health Inspection Institute

weisheng/jiankang health (as in hygiene)/health (as in overall well-being)

wending stable

wenhua shuiping "cultural level," that is, educational level or class

wenjian official document (as from a leader, government agency)

wenming civilized, civilization

wenze zhi responsibility system

wu da weisheng the "Five Hygienes"

xi/xifang the "West"

xiahai "jump into the sea," to jump into the world of business

xianchang "the field," as in doing fieldwork

xiandaihua modernization

xiaoqu gated urban community

xifang guojia Western country

xinku bitter, difficult

xinxian fresh, new

xuanchuan propaganda, information campaign

yimin immigrant

yimin chengshi city of immigrants

yingchou entertainment activities (for example, banqueting)

yingji emergency, urgent

yiqing epidemic outbreak situation

you wenhua "has culture," often used to denote whether someone is educated or "cultured"

yufang weizhu "prevention first"

yufang yixue preventive medicine

zhanzhu zheng temporary residence permit

zhengchang normal

zhengfu government

zhiliang/suzhi quality of a thing/quality of a person

zhiye weisheng occupational hygiene/occupational health

zhongyi Traditional Chinese Medicine

zhongzhuan vocational high school

zhongguo meng China Dream

zhuanjia experts

zhuanye renyuan professionals, specialists

zhuren director

Notes

INTRODUCTION

1. The Ministry of Health (MOH) in 2013 merged with the State Family Planning Commission to form the National Health and Family Planning Commission (NHFPC). In this book I will continue to refer to the MOH, as it was called at the time of my research.

2. All names in this book are pseudonyms, with the exception of nationally or globally recognizable public figures. Certain identifying details of my sources and their institutions, and certain details about the projects they were working on, have been changed for the purposes of protecting confidentiality.

3. This book focuses on urban public health as practiced in government-affiliated, nonclinical public health work units. For the most part I do not examine public health nongovernmental organizations (NGOs), which were few in number and relatively noninfluential in urban southeastern China in the late 2000s. NGOs appear in this book only in the context of their collaborations with the work units studied (see Chapter Two and the Conclusion).

4. Tianmai had an estimated 16 million people as of 2010. By the time I returned in 2014, the estimated population had risen to 20 million.

5. Following my Chinese informants, I use the terms *Western* and *the West* throughout this book to denote the countries of North America, Western Europe, and Australia. Though many scholars have rejected these terms in favor of "Global North," I found it more appropriate in this case to use the terms that my informants used (*xifang*, or *xifang guojia—the West* or *Western countries*).

6. Most older TM CDC members obtained training in the Five Hygienes in a secondary or postsecondary vocational school (*zhongzhuan* or *dazhuan*) program, although bachelor's and master's programs in sanitation-related topics also began proliferating after SARS as public health careers grew in popularity.

7. Sparrows were later replaced by cockroaches as the fourth pest; Rogaski describes variations on the campaign that targeted five pests, including bedbugs (2004).

8. Chinese representatives presented the successes of barefoot doctors at WHO's Alma Ata conference as evidence that "Health for All by the Year 2000" through community involvement, a focus on prevention and basic care, and the use of paraprofessionals, was an attainable goal (Cueto 2004). However, praise for barefoot doctors has over the years been neither universal nor static. Rosenthal (1987), for example, questioned the effectiveness of the undertrained doctors and the success of the overall system.

9. A new health care reform plan that the central government unveiled in 2009 promised to extend health insurance to 90 percent of Chinese, to expand government payments for medications, to reinvest in primary health care through the expansion of community health service centers, to reform the hospital system, to better integrate the public health and clinical care systems, and to invest even more heavily in the public health system (Chen 2009; PRC Ministry of Health 2009a; Hsiao and Hu 2011). These reforms were still in progress as of this writing and have met with some success, providing at least minimal access to basic health coverage for 95 percent of the Chinese population by 2012—though access for rural-to-urban migrants in their host cities continued to be limited (Blumenthal and Hsiao 2015).

10. The reprofessionalization of medicine and public health was accompanied by a parallel movement to professionalize government employment more broadly (Tomba 2014).

11. By the late 1990s, local AESs had already begun separating out HII functions in preparation for this shift.

12. The Chinese FETP, established in 2001, was a two-year training program run by the U.S. CDC in concert with WHO and the Chinese CDC and Ministry of Health. Trainees spent two months in Beijing taking courses and then were sent to one of several participating CDCs in major Chinese cities to complete a field project. The program also spun out several provincial and city-level FETPs run by local leaders, including one in Tianmai.

13. The new International Health Regulations (IHR), which were already in the process of being revised prior to 2003, replaced older regulations that had listed only a few specific diseases (for example, cholera, yellow fever) as reportable at an international level, leaving out any requirement to report a new disease like SARS (Fidler 2005). In addition to broadening the definition of a reportable disease, the new IHR also allowed for nonstate actors to participate in reporting. This opened the door for WHO to go around the state to obtain information about disease outbreaks inside a country (see Mason in press).

14. Holding variety show performances (*biaoyan*) around holidays is a common part of community building in Chinese work units.

15. The word *qunti*, which I translated literally as *group*, is sometimes translated in public health contexts as *community* or *population*. However, given the par-

ticular meanings of these other terms as I use them in the context of this book, I use the more neutral *group* here.

16. Biomedicine is divided into three branches in China: "clinical medicine" (*linchuang yixue*), "preventive medicine" (*yufang yixue*), and "basic medicine" (*jichu yixue*, that is, laboratory-based sciences). According to a professor of preventive medicine at a large university in Guangzhou, where many of my informants studied, "Basic medicine deals with the micro level, clinical with the individual level, and preventive with the crowd (*renqun*)."

17. This transition was never really complete. In the United States, coalitions of physicians, social workers, bureaucrats, policy makers, and many other stakeholders make up the public health profession (Turnock 2012).

18. Like all technical work units, the TM CDC is affiliated with the state but is not technically part of the state. It acts on behalf of the state, via directives from the corresponding local Bureau of Health (BOH). Their status as state-*affiliated* scientists rather than as state civil servants (*gongwuyuan*) was important to my informants in establishing their identities as "professionals" rather than "bureaucrats."

19. Tianmai's arm of the State Family Planning Commission (SFPC) merged with its BOH in August 2009 to form the Tianmai Health and Family Planning Commission (TM HFPC). In this book I will continue to refer to the TM BOH, as it was called at the time of my research.

20. Wu Yi's use of the term *jiankang* to denote "health" is important to note. The Tianmai BOH and CDC at the time of my research had been steadily replacing the term *weisheng* (often translated as *sanitation* or *hygiene*) in department names, initiatives, and campaigns, with the term *jiankang*, which also means "health," but in the broader sense of "well-being" (see Rogaski 2004). Focusing on "health" rather than on "hygiene" shifted the target of public health from the environment in which people lived to the biological bodies of the people themselves.

21. Cho quotes one of her interlocutors telling her the exact same thing (see Cho 2013, 88).

22. Though both *common* and the related term *commons* can in other contexts refer to shared land or other resources, here I use *common* to refer instead to a segment of society expected to benefit from public health measures—that is, the *common* indexed by the term *common good*. The *common* as I use it here is not to be confused with *commons*, which in recent anthropological literature has usually referred to shared property of either a concrete or abstract variety (for example, *biomedical commons*; see Waldby and Mitchell 2006; Reddy 2007). See Wagner (2012) for an overview of recent scholarly treatments of the "commons."

23. Until 2013, when the State Family Planning Commission merged with the MOH, the family planning program was run through a separate "line" of governance and was not considered to be part of "public health." Note that the one-child policy was amended in October 2015 to allow all families to have two children.

24. These ten departments were: parasitology and molecular biology, HIV/ AIDS, HIV/AIDS laboratory, microbiology, infectious disease, vaccination, food hygiene, environmental hygiene, school hygiene, and outpatient clinic (see Appendix 1).

25. Through the extensive connections that I built up throughout the Pearl River Delta region during the course of my fieldwork I eventually was able to gain limited access to the GZ CDC and other Guangzhou institutions, though never to the extent that I did in Tianmai.

CHAPTER ONE

1. Portions of this chapter appeared in altered form in Katherine A. Mason, 2012, "Mobile Migrants, Mobile Germs: Migration, Contagion and Boundary-Building in Shenzhen, China after SARS." *Medical Anthropology: Cross-Cultural Studies in Health and Illness* 31(2): 113–131.

2. When I returned for follow-up fieldwork in 2014, total population estimates had reached 20 million, with the percentage of floating population approximately the same.

3. In 2014 the central government announced plans to move toward a national residency registration system (*jumin hukou*), which would eliminate the general rural–urban distinction and provide greater access to *hukou*s for migrants to small and medium (but not large) cities by 2020.

4. Since 1988 those with a rural *hukou* could legally work in Tianmai if they registered with the local authorities and obtained a "temporary residence permit" (*zhanzhu zheng*) and if their employers paid a fee (Zhang 2001; Ngai 2005). As of August 2008, properly registered and employed migrants in Tianmai were able to apply for "permanent residence cards" and occasionally could enter lotteries or accumulate "points" to obtain urban *hukou*. Still, a large number of migrants continued to fail to register for the reasons discussed in the text.

5. See Markel (1997) for similar differentiations between desirable and undesirable nineteenth-century American immigrants.

6. An estimated 30 million people died during the famines and violence associated with the Great Leap Forward (1958–1961), when Chairman Mao rapidly communized villages and pushed peasants to boost production to impossible levels (see Becker 1997).

7. In some migrant-dense areas, local governments institutionalized this distinction between true residents and *liudong renkou* through the creation of "floating population rental management bureaus" (*liudong renkou chuzuwu guanli suo*) at the "street" (*jiedao*) level of local government. These rental management bureaus functioned as what one informant called "residents' committees for the floating population."

8. Some of the villages were also converted into *xiaoqu*s for wealthier Tianmai residents.

9. Tomba (2014) suggests that low-income, low-*suzhi* residents of urban areas are more easily reached by local governments due to the reach of *shequ*s ("communities"), the lowest level of administrative governance, which often has trouble reaching into the self-governing *xiaoqu*s. I found that migrants were in some ways just as insulated from the power of the municipal government as wealthier *xiaoqu*s were, for the reasons stated in the text.

10. Mandarin (*putonghua*) is the official national language of the PRC and the lingua franca for most immigrants to Tianmai.

11. According to several young professionals in other fields whom I knew in this part of China, tougher economic times and a more competitive business climate had been leading to a rise in applications to government *danwei*s among educated youth in recent years. Tomba observed the same trend in his research on middle-class urban neighborhoods in China in which "after years in the doldrums, public employment has again become a top preference among job seekers" (2014, 115). Part of the appeal was rapidly rising salaries in the public sector, which, combined with strong welfare benefits, made government jobs competitive with private-sector jobs once again. TM CDC employees, however, still complained that their salaries were paltry compared with their peers who worked for corporations. For them, by far the biggest draw of a government job was its stability (*wending*).

12. As a foreign anthropologist, I was able to penetrate this insular community only by first gaining the trust of the *danwei*'s highest leader. Once I had entered the *danwei*, whenever anyone questioned who I was or why I was present at a particular event, my colleagues would simply state, "She is of our *danwei*" (*ta shi women danwei de*), and the matter would be dropped.

13. Implemented in December 2003, this program guarantees free counseling and testing for HIV as well as free antiretroviral drugs to rural and poor urban residents who test HIV positive and have a CD4 count below 200, free drugs to prevent transmission from mother to child (PMTCT), free education for AIDS orphans, and care for people living with HIV/AIDS. In Tianmai, all pregnant women and their partners, regardless of migration status, had access to free drugs through the PMTCT program. Other HIV-positive migrants without *hukou* normally could not obtain free drugs in Tianmai.

14. This is the same argument that has been made in the United States, for example, to explain why undocumented immigrants should not have access to health services (King 2007).

15. Although official policies to deport rural migrants from cities ended in 2003, unregistered rural-to-urban migrants still faced fines and harassment by police at the time of my research.

16. By mid-2010, most city- and district-level disease control institutions in Tianmai had ceased conducting physical exams, turning the task over to hospital

clinics and street-level CDCs. At the time of my fieldwork in 2008 and 2009, however, clinics still provided much of the income for local CDCs.

17. The clinic workers rarely acknowledged the fact that many members of the floating population spoke Mandarin poorly and thus may have had language barriers to understanding what was being asked of them.

18. An important exception to this is the work that the HIV/AIDS department did. The implications of this exception will be explored in the Conclusion.

CHAPTER TWO

1. On World AIDS Day 2003, then-Premier Wen Jiabao publicly shook hands with several AIDS patients in a move intended to signal a greater commitment to HIV/AIDS control in China and to reduce stigma (Liu and Kaufman 2006).

2. Street-level (*jiedao*) CDCs were established in two districts of Tianmai in 2002 and 2003. Prior to that, all lower-level public health institutions (vaccination stations, community health centers, and so on) were overseen by hospital *fangbao kes*. The *jiedao* CDCs were distinct from the other levels in that they incorporated the functions of the Health Inspection Institute as well as the CDC functions, thus more resembling the old AESs. Community health service centers represented the lowest level of both public health and clinical care and the place where these two "lines" of the health care system met.

3. The "technical direction" that higher-level CDCs were supposed to give to lower levels included running citywide conferences, offering scientific training to the lower levels, and assisting with initiatives. In addition, higher-level CDCs delegated responsibilities to the lower levels during citywide campaigns or emergency responses and were in charge of running the city's surveillance systems.

4. According to WHO (Ma et al. 2014), measles cases in China did steadily decline between 2008 and 2012, hitting an all-time low in 2012 of approximately 6,100 cases. This number rose rapidly in the several years following 2012, with both Chinese and foreign officials blaming the rise largely on migrant workers who failed to vaccinate their children (see also Zhuang 2014).

5. Tomba (2014) notes that in large cities many residents committees (*juweihui*) were reorganized into *shequ* committees by the 2000s. I found in my fieldwork that both names were used interchangeably, with *juweihui* continuing to be used most often.

6. Note that as the upper-level CDCs had no administrative power over the lower-level CDCs; they could not repay them with a better job, better salary, or the like. It is precisely this lack of direct influence over the lower levels that made *guanxi*-building so important.

7. Note that the purchase of sex was rarely involved in the *yingchou* activities I observed. This is not to say that soliciting of prostitutes or participation in the kinds of sexually charged karaoke sessions that other scholars have described never

occurred, but, to the extent that it did, it was outside the normal domain of *guanxi* building at the *danwei*s with which I worked (see Uretsky 2008; Mason 2013).

8. Factories were also inspected, but in Tianmai the Occupational Health Institute conducted these inspections at the city level.

9. Unlike the former AES, the TM CDC did not have the power to issue fines—it could only pass on a report to the Health Inspection Institute.

10. Notably, my informants saw building *guanxi* as less necessary in the case of mess halls and lower-end restaurants, which were charged lower prices and visited less often and therefore were seen as bearing a smaller burden. One might assume these places might be more likely to have sanitation problems, and I often witnessed desperate efforts on the part of these lower-end places to build *guanxi* or to outright bribe the inspectors. The inspectors always rebuffed these attempts.

11. The Tianmai city budget office in 2009 promised to make *chuangshou* unnecessary by providing "*quanbu bokuan*," or "complete funding allocation," for the TM CDC by late 2010. As a stipulation of *quanbu bokuan*, the CDC would no longer be authorized to raise money on its own. Paid inspections were to be "canceled" (*quxiao*) through a phasing-out program. Similar shifts took place across the Pearl River Delta. A return visit to Tianmai in 2014, however, revealed that some sanitation inspections were still being conducted.

12. Guo quickly clarified that those who "*duguo shu*" could include people with vocational education as well and that the *really* uneducated workers were those who had finished only a standard junior high or high school education. At the time that she began her education, vocational school was still the highest form of education available; with universities closed by the tumult of the Cultural Revolution until the late 1970s, bachelor's degrees did not become widely accessible until much later.

13. In 1997, the central government passed a law standardizing professional requirements for health practitioners; this was followed in 2001 with the establishment of the NHPSQE (NHPSQE Expert Committee 2009). Aspiring professionals could test at the elementary (*chuji*), middle (*zhongji*), or high (*gaoji*) levels. Those entering local public health institutions had to pass both the national civil servant exam and the new exam, though these rules were often bent based on *guanxi*. The version of the exam that public health professionals took tested in the areas of disease control (*jibing kongzhi*, including epidemiology, biostatistics, and some laboratory sciences), public hygiene (*gonggong weisheng*), occupational hygiene (*zhiye weisheng*), maternal and child health (*fuyou baojian*), and health education (*jiankang jiaoyu*). Students in undergraduate medical colleges who majored in preventive medicine studied these topics in their final year of school, following four years of basic science and clinical training (undergraduate medical degrees in China are five-year programs).

14. See Mason 2013 for a discussion of the gendered aspects of this issue.

15. These debates over the importance of sanitation and other environmental factors to health call to mind long-standing debates in the history of Western public health (Ackerknecht 1948; McKeown and Brown 1955; Rosen 1993; Hamlin 1998).

16. In the summer of 2008, several milk processing factories in China were found to be adding melamine, a plastic additive, to baby formula and other milk products to artificially raise the measured protein content of their products. By November 2008 approximately 300,000 people had been affected, six infants had died from kidney damage, and another 860 babies had been hospitalized.

17. Local Tianmai laws were even stricter than the national laws passed in the wake of the outbreak (China Standing Committee of the National People's Congress 2004).

18. When it came to a new type of influenza, as well as malaria, dengue fever, rabies, or a resurgence of SARS, a single case qualified as a *yiqing*. But the situation was murkier when it came to lower-profile diseases. What qualified as an "epidemic situation" depended in part on written regulations (national, provincial, and city), in part on the discretion or skittishness of local *danwei* leaders, and in part on regulations put in place by the city CDC. National regulations, for example, defined a *yiqing* of ordinary influenza as twenty clustered cases, Guangdong defined it as fifteen, and Tianmai as only five cases. Usually an investigation involved taking a team of people to the hospital to visit the affected patients and to conduct a survey to try to determine how, when, and where they were exposed. Investigators then visited contacts and gave instructions to contacts, local hospitals and CDCs for how to monitor for disease symptoms.

19. The city CDC also directly investigated all cases of HIV/AIDS in pregnant women or new mothers, as well as all food poisoning cases reported in restaurants registered with the city CDC.

20. According to birth planning regulations, urban residents ordinarily were limited to one child per family, and rural residents to up to two children depending on the circumstances. A policy change announced in late 2013 liberalized the rule to allow couples in which either partner is a single child him- or herself to have two children, and another major policy change in 2015 transformed the one-child policy into a two-child-for-all policy. Female migrant workers were often accused of coming to the city to illicitly bear extra children.

CHAPTER THREE

1. *Keti*, which translates literally as "problem" or "research question," refers to a wide variety of projects that involve some element of research—ranging from the testing of a new HIV counseling intervention, to an epidemiological research project to study measles prevalence, to a molecular biology project that seeks to identify genes that predispose individuals to having a stroke. The term sometimes

also refers to the grant to which one would apply to fund such a project. *Keyan* usually refers more specifically to academic research, or to the content of a *keti*, though at the institutions where I did my research the two terms often were used interchangeably.

2. Award amounts were scaled according to the SCI (Science Citation Index) ranking of the journal in which the article was published. Journals with the highest rankings (like *Nature* and *Science*) earned 10,000 RMB, whereas journals in a midlevel ranking (a well-respected specialized journal, for example) would earn perhaps 5,000 RMB.

3. This is a charge commonly made about Chinese work in all areas, particularly creative works (Alford 1995; Mertha 2005) as well as science (Cao 2004; Poo 2004).

4. For example, in a famous case that Petryna cites, U.S. researchers conducted a clinical trial in Uganda in 1994 to test the effectiveness of a short-course AZT treatment for the prevention of mother-to-child transmission of HIV. Research participants on the control arm of the study received a placebo rather than the AZT treatment that was the standard of care in the United States. Researchers defended their decision by arguing that giving a placebo was ethical in Uganda even if it would not be in the United States because the standard of care in Uganda was to receive no medication at all (Rothman 2000; Petryna 2005).

5. Medical schools first introduced medical ethics as a subject in the 1980s, but at that point what was taught mostly took the form of applied socialist ethics (Hsiao and Hu 2011). In the 1990s medical ethics courses broadened and became mandatory.

6. This may be a misreading of Confucian teachings, which suggest not that the virtuous person does whatever he or she would want to have done to him- or herself but rather that he or she is obliged to do certain things for another person based on the nature of the interpersonal relationship at hand (see Tu 1979; Yao 2000).

7. This slippage can be seen in other contexts as well. For example, Sankar (2004) writes about the "therapeutic misconception," in which patients mistakenly believe when providing informed consent that they are agreeing to receive a treatment, rather than agreeing to serve as research subjects. Sankar argues that researchers sometimes encourage this misconception through the manner in which they present the information. In addition, in the age of electronic medical records (EMR), researchers more and more often are mining large amounts of data that were originally gathered to aid in clinical care (Ioannidis 2013).

8. The informed consent forms also promised the workers access to the results of their blood tests, but the factory bosses usually were the ones who received the entire group's results and effectively had discretion to decide how, and whether, to distribute them.

9. Note that the value of the free checkup should be taken in the context of the scarcity of access to health services available to the floating population, as detailed in Chapter One.

10. It is unlikely that the migrants felt any more free to refuse to participate in the blood donation drive than in this blood draw—see Jing (2011) on the coercive nature of "voluntary" blood drives in China.

11. Many thanks to an anonymous reviewer for pointing this out.

12. This is a good example of how "the masses" differed from "the population" (see Introduction and Chapter Two). Among the masses, there should be no normal distributional curve to describe group characteristics—everyone is supposed to be exactly the same, and so any measurable value should be the same across the board. Populations, on the other hand, exhibit qualities that can and often do range quite widely across a distribution—implying the importance of individual variation, if not necessarily agency. This may be one reason why *xuanchuan*, developed for the purposes of manipulating the masses, seemed to do a poor job of manipulating the population.

13. During my fieldwork I spent a total of about two months, in increments from several days to several weeks, working with students at the public health school at Jiang's university. My goals were to understand how the highly educated recruits who were changing the face of the TM CDC were being trained.

14. Stories about this type of fraud appeared in newspapers on a regular basis.

15. In a paper criticizing this proposal, bioethicists Rothstein and Shoben (2013) dispute whether consent bias is really as important a source of error as the IOM and others contend.

CHAPTER FOUR

1. Portions of this chapter appeared in altered form in Katherine A. Mason, 2010. "Becoming Modern after SARS: Battling H1N1 and the Politics of Backwardness in China's Pearl River Delta." Special Issue, "Epidemic Orders." *Behemoth—A Journal on Civilisation* 2010(3): 8–35.

2. The index case was said to have had contact with civets in a wet market prior to getting ill. Civets were later shown to be victims rather than perpetrators: Apparently the virus passed from humans to civets rather than vice versa (Janies et al. 2008).

3. An updated WHO plan published in April 2009 changed the meaning of phase 5 to be essentially the same as the pandemic phase and removed the recommendation for efforts to delay transmission during this phase, though it retained recommendations for exit and entry screening (WHO 2009). At the time of the outbreak, my informants did not seem to be familiar with the new plan.

4. This interviewee proved prescient. In late 2014, during the height of the West African Ebola epidemic and shortly after the first Ebola case was diagnosed

in the United States, several U.S. states declared mandatory quarantines of anyone returning from West Africa who had had direct contact with an Ebola patient—regardless of symptoms. The strong resistance and outcry that accompanied the quarantining of an initial test case in New Jersey—a young nurse who had been treating Ebola patients in Sierra Leone—indicated just how dire the threat would have to be to expand such a program.

5. Theresa MacPhail's account of H1N1 quarantines in Hong Kong (2014) similarly suggested that that territory's cultural acceptance and governance structure contributed to a sense among Hong Kongers that quarantine was uniquely suited to Hong Kong.

CONCLUSION

1. Ironically, the event concluded with a raucous banquet in which the recovering drug addicts were pressured to vigorously toast (with copious amounts of whiskey) the city public health leaders who had helped them.

2. Although my informants recognized that many chronic diseases (for example, diabetes) had social components as well, foreign funding and support for addressing these problems was sparser, and the influence of the biosocial approach to intervention was more limited. Most chronic disease initiatives in Tianmai and Guangzhou consisted of traditional exercises in distributing propaganda to large numbers of people at once, often at public fairs dedicated to this purpose. In addition, chronic diseases were understood to be diseases of wealth and thus not thought to significantly affect the floating population or other vulnerable or stigmatized populations.

3. Anyone regardless of residency status could come to the TM CDC clinic for free testing and counseling.

4. Health-related NGOs in Tianmai were sparse and in most cases could operate legally only in collaboration with a local CDC. Most health NGOs did HIV/AIDS work, and Chu's project was one of only a couple of TM CDC-NGO collaborations that I observed being active during my fieldwork.

Bibliography

Abrams, Herbert K. 2001. "The Resurgence of Sexually Transmitted Disease in China." *Journal of Public Health Policy* 22(4): 429–440.

Acheson, Roy M., and Elizabeth Fee. 1991. "Introduction." In *A History of Education in Public Health: Health that Mocks the Doctor's Rules*. Edited by Elizabeth Fee and Roy M. Acheson, 1–14. New York: Oxford University Press.

Ackerknecht, Erwin H. 1948. "Anticontagionism between 1821 and 1867." *Bulletin of the History of Medicine* 22: 562–593.

Adams, Vincanne. 2013. "Evidence-Based Global Public Health: Subjects, Profits, Erasures." In *When People Come First: Critical Studies in Global Health*. Edited by Joao Biehl and Adriana Petryna. Princeton, NJ: Princeton University Press.

Ai Ming 2003. "Rethinking SARS: Socioeconomic Development and Health Education" [*Fansi SARS: Shehui Jingji Fazhan yu Jiankang Jiaoyu*]. *China Journal of Health Education* [*Zhongguo Jiankang Jiaoyu*] 19(7): 477–479.

Alford, William P. 1995. *To Steal a Book Is an Elegant Offense: Intellectual Property Law in Chinese Civilization*. Stanford, CA: Stanford University Press.

Alford, William P., and Kenneth Winston. 2011. "Introduction." In *Prospects for the Professions in China*. Edited by William P. Alford, Kenneth Winston, and William Kirby, 1–21. New York: Routledge.

Althusser, Louis. 1971. Ideology and Ideological State Apparatuses. *In Lenin and Philosophy and Other Essays*. Translated by Ben Brewster. 127–186. New York: Monthly Review Press.

Anagnost, Ann. 1997. *National Past-Times: Narrative, Representation, and Power in Modern China*. Durham, NC: Duke University Press.

———. 2004. "The Corporeal Politics of Quality (Suzhi)." *Public Culture* 16(2): 189–208.

Anderson, Benedict R. 1991 [1983]. *Imagined Communities: Reflections on the Origins and Spread of Nationalism*. London: Verso.

Bach, Jonathan. 2010. "'They Come in Peasants and Leave Citizens': Urban Villages and the Making of Shenzhen, China." *Cultural Anthropology* 25(3): 421–458.

Barnes, David S. 1995. *The Making of a Social Disease: Tuberculosis in Nineteenth-Century France.* Berkeley: University of California Press.

———. 2006. *The Great Stink of Paris and the Nineteenth-Century Struggle against Filth and Germs.* Baltimore, MD: Johns Hopkins University Press.

Bayer, Ronald, and Amy L. Fairchild. 2004. "The Genesis of Public Health Ethics." *Bioethics* 18(6): 475–492.

Beauchamp, Tom L., and James F. Childress. 2009. *Principles of Biomedical Ethics*, sixth edition. New York: Oxford University Press.

Becker, Jasper. 1997. *Hungry Ghosts: Mao's Secret Famine.* New York: The Free Press.

Benjamin, Walter. 1969. "The Work of Art in the Age of Mechanical Reproduction." In *Illuminations: Essays and Reflections.* Edited by Hannah Arendt, translated by Harry Zohn, 217–252. Berlin: Schocken.

Benton, Adia. 2014. "The Epidemic Will be Militarized: Watching Outbreak as the West African Ebola Epidemic Unfolds." Fieldsights—Hot Spots, *Cultural Anthropology Online*, October 7.

———. 2015. *HIV Exceptionalism: Development through Disease in Sierra Leone.* Minneapolis: Minnesota University Press.

Berdahl, Daphne. 1999. *Where the World Ended: Re-unification and Identity in the German Borderland.* Berkeley: University of California Press.

Biehl, Joao. 2005. *Vita: Life in a Zone of Social Abandonment.* Berkeley: University of California Press.

Biehl, Joao, and Adriana Petryna, eds. 2013. *When People Come First: Critical Studies in Global Health.* Princeton, NJ: Princeton University Press.

Bingham, Nick, and Steve Hinchliffe. 2008. "Mapping the Multiplicities of Biosecurity." In *Biosecurity Interventions: Global Health and Security in Question.* Edited by Andrew Lakoff and Stephen J. Collier, 173–194. New York: Columbia University Press.

Blum, Susan Debra. 2007. *Lies That Bind: Chinese Truth, Other Truths.* New York: Rowman and Littlefield.

Blumenthal, David, and William Hsiao. 2015. "Lessons from the East—China's Rapidly Evolving Health Care System." *New England Journal of Medicine* 372(14): 1281–1285.

Bosk, Charles L. 1981. *Forgive and Remember: Managing Medical Failure.* Chicago: University of Chicago Press.

Brandt, Allan M. 1978. "Racism and Research: The Case of the Tuskegee Syphilis Study." *Hastings Center Report* 8(6): 21–29.

Brandt, Allan M., and Martha Gardner. 2000. "Antagonism and Accommodation: Interpreting the Relationship between Public Health and Medicine in the United States during the 20th Century." *American Journal of Public Health* 90(5): 707–715.

Bray, David. 2006. "Building 'Community': New Strategies of Governance in Urban China." *Economy and Society* 35(4): 530–549.

Briggs, Charles L., and Clara Mantini-Briggs. 2003. *Stories in the Time of Cholera: Racial Profiling during a Medical Nightmare.* Berkeley: University of California Press.

Brown, Hannah. 2015. "Global Health Partnerships, Governance, and Sovereign Responsibility in Western Kenya." *American Ethnologist* 42(2): 340–355.

Buch, Elena. 2013. "Senses of Care: Embodying Inequality and Sustaining Personhood in the Home Care of Older Adults in Chicago." *American Ethnologist* 40(4): 637–650.

Burchell, Graham, Colin Gordon, and Peter Miller, eds. 1991. *The Foucault Effect: Studies in Governmentality.* Chicago: University of Chicago Press.

Caduff, Carlo. 2014. "On the Verge of Death: Visions of Biological Vulnerability." *Annual Review of Anthropology* 43: 105–121.

Canguilhem, Georges. 1991 [1978]. *The Normal and the Pathological.* Translated by C. R. Fawcett with R. S. Cohen. New York: Zone Books.

Cao, Cong. 2004. "Chinese Science and the 'Nobel Prize Complex.'" *Minerva* 42(2): 151–172.

Cao, Cong, and Richard P. Suttmeier. 2001. "China's New Scientific Elite: Distinguished Young Scientists, the Research Environment and Hopes for Chinese Science." *China Quarterly* 168: 960–984.

Carey, Benedict. 2015. "Study on Attitudes towards Same-Sex Marriage Is Retracted by a Scientific Journal." *New York Times,* May 28.

Carpenter, Daniel P. 2010. *Reputation and Power: Organizational Image and Pharmaceutical Regulation at the FDA.* Princeton, NJ: Princeton University Press.

Castaneda, Heide. 2010. "Deportation Deferred: 'Illegality,' Visibility, and Recognition in Contemporary Germany." In *The Deportation Regime: Sovereignty, Space, and the Freedom of Movement.* Edited by Nicholas De Genova and Nathalie Mae Peutz, 245–261. Durham, NC: Duke University Press.

Chan, Kam Wing, and Li Zhang. 1999. "The Hukou System and Rural–Urban Migration in China: Processes and Changes." *China Quarterly* (160): 818–855.

Chan, Margaret. 2007. "Health Diplomacy in the 21st Century." Address to Directorate for Health and Social Affairs, Oslo, February 13.

Chen, C. C. 1989. *Medicine in Rural China: A Personal Account.* Berkeley: University of California Press.

Chen Zheng, Xu Wenzhong, and Tan Jiadi. 2004. "Using 'Build a Healthy City' as a Way to Improve Local Public Health" [*Yi Jianshe Jiankang Chengshi Zaiti Tongchou Tigao Chengxiang Gonggong Weisheng Shuiping*]. *China Journal of Public Health Management* [*Zhongguo Gonggong Weisheng Guanli*] 20(5): 403–405.

Chen, Zhu. 2009. "Launch of the Health-Care Reform Plan in China." *The Lancet* 373(9672): 1322–1324.

China Standing Committee of the National People's Congress. 2004. "Law of the People's Republic of China on the Prevention and Treatment of Infectious Diseases" [*Zhonghua Renmin Gongheguo Chuanranbing Fangzhi Fa*]. Retrieved on April 6, 2011, from http://vip.chinalawinfo.com/NewLaw2002/SLC/SLC.asp?Db=chl&Gid=54998.

Cho, Mun Young. 2013. *The Specter of "The People": Urban Poverty in the Northeast of China*. Ithaca, NY: Cornell University Press.

Cohen, Myron S., Gao Ping, Kim Fox, and Gail E. Henderson. 2000. "Sexually Transmitted Diseases in the People's Republic of China in Y2K: Back to the Future." *Sexually Transmitted Diseases* 27(3): 143–145.

Cook, Ian G., and Trevor J. B. Dummer. 2004. "Changing Health in China: Re-Evaluating the Epidemiological Transition Model." *Health Policy* 67(3): 329–343.

Coughlin, Steven S. 2006. "Ethical Issues in Epidemiologic Research and Public Health Practice." *Emerging Themes in Epidemiology* 3(16).

Crane, Johanna Tayloe. 2013. *Scrambling for Africa: AIDS, Expertise, and the Rise of American Global Health Science*. Ithaca, NY: Cornell University Press.

Cribb, Alan. 2009. "Why Ethics? What Kind of Ethics for Public Health?" In *Public Health Ethics and Practice*. Edited by Stephen Peckham and Alison Hann, 17–32. Portland, OR: The Policy Press.

Csordas, Thomas J. 1993. "Somatic Modes of Attention." *Cultural Anthropology* 8(2): 135–156.

Cueto, Marcos. 2004. "The Origins of Primary Health Care and Selective Primary Health Care." *American Journal of Public Health* 94(11): 1864–1874.

Das, Venna. 2000. "The Act of Witnessing: Violence, Poisonous Knowledge, and Subjectivity." In *Violence and Subjectivity*. Edited by Veena Das, Arthur Kleinman, Mamphela Ramphele, and Pamela Reynolds, 205–225. Berkeley: University of California Press.

Datta, Jessica, and Allan S. Kessell. 2009. "Unlinked Anonymous Blood Testing for Public Health Purposes: An Ethical Dilemma?" In *Public Health Ethics and Practice*. Edited by Stephen Peckham and Alison Hann, 101–116. Portland, OR: The Policy Press.

De Genova, Nicholas P. 2002. "Migrant 'Illegality' and Deportability in Everyday Life." *Annual Review of Anthropology* 31: 419–447.

Derksen, Linda. 2000. "Towards a Sociology of Measurement: The Meaning of Measurement Error in the Case of DNA Profiling." *Social Studies of Science* 30(6): 803–845.

Devisch, Ignaas. 2013. *Jean-Luc Nancy and the Question of Community*. New York: Bloomsbury.

Dikotter, Frank. 1992. *The Discourse of Race in Modern China*. Stanford, CA: Stanford University Press.

Dong, Zigang, Christian W. Hoven, and Allen Rosenfield. 2005. "Lessons from the Past: Poverty and Market Forces Combine to Keep Rural China Unhealthy." *Nature* 433: 573–574.

Douglas, Mary. 2002 [1966]. *Purity and Danger: An Analysis of Concepts of Pollution and Taboo*. New York: Routledge Classics.

Durkheim, Emile. 1992 [1957]. *Professional Ethics and Civic Morals*. Translated by C. Brookfield. New York: Routledge.

Epstein, Steven. 2007. *Inclusion: The Politics of Difference in Medical Research*. Chicago: University of Chicago Press.

Fan, C. Cindy. 2008. *China on the Move: Migration, the State, and the Household*. New York: Routledge.

Fanon, Frantz. 1986. *Black Skin, White Masks*. Translated by C. L. Markman. London: Pluto Press.

Farmer, Paul. 1999. *Infections and Inequalities: The Modern Plagues*. Berkeley: University of California Press.

———. 2003. *Pathologies of Power: Health, Human Rights, and the New War on the Poor*. Berkeley: University of California Press.

Farmer, Paul, Arthur Kleinman, Jim Yong Kim, and Matthew Basilico, eds. 2013. *Reimagining Global Health: An Introduction*. Berkeley: University of California Press.

Farquhar, Judith. 2002. *Appetites: Food and Sex in Postsocialist China*. Durham, NC: Duke University Press.

Fei Xiaotong. 1980 [1939]. *Peasant Life in China: A Field Study of Country Life in the Yangtse Valley*. London and Henley: Routledge and Kegan Paul.

———. 1992 [1948]. *From the Soil: The Foundations of Chinese Society*. Translated by G. G. Hamilton and W. Zheng. Berkeley: University of California Press.

Ferguson, James. 1994. *The Anti-Politics Machine: Development, Depoliticization, and Bureaucratic Power in Lesotho*. Minneapolis: University of Minnesota Press.

———. 1999. *Expectations of Modernity: Myths and Meanings of Urban Life on the Zambian Copperbelt*. Berkeley: University of California Press.

Fidler, David P. 2004. *SARS, Governance and the Globalization of Disease*. New York: Palgrave Macmillan.

———. 2005. "From International Sanitary Conventions to Global Health Security: The New International Health Regulations." *Chinese Journal of International Law* 4(2): 325–392.

Fleck, Ludwik. 1979. *Genesis and Development of a Scientific Fact*. Chicago: University of Chicago Press.

Flory, James, and Ezekiel Emanuel. 2004. "Interventions to Improve Research Participants' Understanding in Informed Consent for Research." *Journal of the American Medical Association* 292(13): 1593–1601.

Fong, Vanessa L. 2007. "Morality, Cosmopolitanism, or Academic Achievement? Discourses on 'Quality' and Urban Chinese-Only-Children's Claims to Ideal Personhood." *City and Society* 19(1): 86–113.

———. 2010. *Paradise Redefined: Transnational Chinese Students and the Quest for Flexible Citizenship in the Developed World*. Stanford, CA: Stanford University Press.

Fong, Vanessa L., and Rachel Murphy. 2006. *Chinese Citizenship: Views from the Margins*. New York: Routledge.

Foster, Drew. 2015. "Will Academia Waste the Michael LaCour Scandal?" *New York*, June 5.

Foucault, Michael. 1989 [1973]. *The Birth of the Clinic: An Archaeology of Medical Perception*. Translated by A. M. Sheridan. New York: Routledge.

———. 1990 [1976]. *The History of Sexuality, vol. 1: An Introduction*. Translated by R. Hurley. New York: Vintage Books.

Franklin, Sarah. 1995. "Postmodern Procreation: A Cultural Account of Assisted Reproduction." In *Conceiving the New World Order: The Global Politics of Reproduction*. Edited by Faye Ginsburg and Rayna Rapp, 323–345. Berkeley: University of California Press.

Fried, Linda, Michael J. Klag, Julio J. Frenk, Harrison C. Specer, Margaret E. Bentley, Pierre Buekens, and Donald S. Burke. 2010. "Global Health Is Public Health." *Lancet* 375(9714): 535–537.

Fukuyama, Francis. 1995. *Trust: The Social Virtues and the Creation of Prosperity*. New York: Free Press.

Fullwiley, Duana. 2007. "The Molecularization of Race: Institutionalizing Human Difference in Pharmacogenetics Practice." *Science as Culture* 16(1): 1–30.

———. 2008. "The Biologistical Construction of Race: 'Admixture' Technology and the New Genetic Medicine." *Social Studies of Science* 38(5): 695–735.

Giddens, Anthony. 1990. *The Consequences of Modernity*. Stanford, CA: Stanford University Press.

Gieryn, Thomas F. 2002. "Three Truth Spots." *Journal of History of the Behavioral Sciences* 38(2): 113–132.

Goldade, Kathryn. 2009. "'Health Is Hard Here' or 'Health for All'? The Politics of Blame, Gender, and Health Care for Undocumented Nicaraguan Migrants in Costa Rica." *Medical Anthropology Quarterly* 23(4): 483–503.

Good, Byron. 1994. *Medicine, Rationality, and Experience: An Anthropological Perspective*. Cambridge, UK: Cambridge University Press.

Gostin, Lawrence O. 2002. *Public Health Law and Ethics: A Reader*. Berkeley: University of California Press.

———. 2009. "Influenza A (H1N1) and Pandemic Preparedness Under the Rule of International Law." *Journal of the American Medical Association* 301(22): 2376–2378.

Gostin, Lawrence O., Ronald Bayer, and Amy L. Fairchild. 2003. "Ethical and Legal Challenges Posed by Severe Acute Respiratory Syndrome: Implications for the Control of Severe Infectious Disease Threats." *Journal of the American Medical Association* 290(24): 3229–3237.

Goudsmit, Jaap. 2004. *Viral Fitness: The Next SARS and West Nile in the Making.* New York: Oxford University Press.

Greenhalgh, Susan, and Edwin A. Winckler. 2005. *Governing China's Population: From Leninist to Neoliberal Biopolitics.* Stanford, CA: Stanford University Press.

Greger, Michael. 2006. "Industrial Animal Agriculture's Role in the Emergence and Spread of Disease." In *The Meat Crisis: Developing More Sustainable Production and Consumption.* Edited by Joyce D'Silva and John Webster, 161–172. Washington, DC: Earthscan.

Guo, Jinhua. 2008. *Stigma: Social Suffering for Social Exclusion and Social Insecurity: From the Ethnography of Mental Illness to the Ethnography of HIV/AIDS in China.* PhD dissertation, Department of Anthropology, Harvard University.

Guo, Jinhua, and Arthur Kleinman. 2011. "Stigma: HIV/AIDS, Mental Illness and China's Nonpersons." In *Deep China: The Moral Life of the Person,* 237–262. Berkeley: University of California Press.

Hacking, Ian. 1990. *The Taming of Chance.* Cambridge, UK: Cambridge University Press.

Hamlin, Christopher. 1998. *Public Health and Social Justice in the Age of Chadwick, Britain 1800–1854.* Cambridge, UK: Cambridge University Press.

Harrell, Stevan, ed. 1995. *Cultural Encounters in China's Ethnic Frontiers.* Seattle: University of Washington Press.

Hay, Simon I., Dylan B. George, Catherine L. Moyes, and John S. Brownstein. 2013. "Big Data Opportunities for Global Infectious Disease Surveillance." *PLOS Medicine* 10(4): e1001413.

Hayden, Cori. 2003. *When Nature Goes Public: The Making and Unmaking of Bioprospecting in Mexico.* Princeton, NJ: Princeton University Press.

Hayden, Karen E. 2000. "Stigma and Place: Space, Community, and the Politics of Reputation." *Studies in Symbolic Interaction* 23: 219–239.

He Jiang, Donfeng Gu, Xigui Wu, Kristi Reynolds, Xiufang Duan, Chonghua Yao, Jialiang Wang, Chung-Shiuan Chen, Jing Chen, Rachel P. Wildman, Michael J. Klag, and Paul K. Whelton. 2005. "Major Causes of Death among Men and Women in China." *The New England Journal of Medicine* 353(11): 1124–1134.

Henderson, Gail. 1993. "Physicians in China: Assessing the Impact of Ideology and Organization." In *The Changing Medical Profession: An International Perspective,* edited by Fredric W. Hafferty and John B. McKinlay, 184–196. New York: Oxford University Press.

Henderson, Gail E., Larry R. Churchill, Arlene M. Davis, Michele M. Easter, Christine Grady, Steven Joffe, Nancy Kass, Nancy M. P. King, Charles W.

Lidz, Franklin G. Miller, Daniel K. Nelson, Jeffrey Peppercorn, Barbra B. Rothschild, Pamela Sankar, Benjamin S. Wilfond, and Catherine R. Zimmer. 2007. "Clinical Trials and Medical Care: Defining the Therapeutic Misconception." *PLOS Medicine* 4(11): 1735–1738.

Hershatter, Gail. 1997. *Dangerous Pleasures: Prostitution and Modernity in Twentieth-Century Shanghai.* Berkeley: University of California Press.

Herzfeld, Michael. 1992. *The Social Production of Indifference: Exploring the Symbolic Roots of Western Bureaucracy.* Chicago: University of Chicago Press.

Hess, David J. 1995. *Science and Technology in a Multicultural World: The Cultural Politics of Facts and Artifacts.* New York: Columbia University Press.

Hoffman, Lisa M. 2010. *Patriotic Professionalism in Urban China: Fostering Talent.* Philadelphia: Temple University Press.

Hong H. 2009. "Scared to Death by SARS" *[Bei SARS Xiasi].* Southern Metropolis *Weekly [Nandu Zhoukan],* May 22, 35–36.

Horn, Joshua S. 1969. *Away with All the Pests: An English Surgeon in People's China.* New York: Paul Hamlyn.

Horton, Sarah, and Judith C. Barker. 2009. "'Stains' on Their Self-Discipline: Public Health, Hygiene, and the Disciplining of Undocumented Immigrant Parents in the Nation's Internal Borderlands." *American Ethnologist* 36(4): 784–798.

Hsiao, William C. 1995. "The Chinese Health Care System: Lessons for Other Nations." *Social Science and Medicine* 41(8): 1047–1055.

Hsiao, William C., and Linying Hu. 2011. "The State of Medical Professionalism in China: Past, Present, and Future." In *Prospects for the Professions in China.* Edited by W. P. Alford, K. Winston, and W. C. Kirby, 111–128. New York: Routledge.

Hu Runhua. 2003. "Brief Discussion of the Meaning of 'Public Health'" *[Qiantan Gonggong Weisheng de Hanyi]. Chinese Medical Research Management Journal [Zhonghua Yiliao Keyan Guanli Zazhi]* 16(3): 133–135.

Hwang, Kwang-kuo. 1987. "Face and Favor: The Chinese Power Game." *The American Journal of Sociology* 92(4): 944–974.

Hyde, Sandra Teresa. 2007. *Eating Spring Rice: The Cultural Politics of AIDS in Southwest China.* Berkeley: University of California Press.

Ikels, Charlotte, ed. 2004. *Filial Piety: Practice and Discourse in Contemporary East Asia.* Stanford, CA: Stanford University Press.

Illich, Ivan. 1975. *Medical Nemesis: The Expropriation of Health Care.* London: Calder and Boyars.

IOM (Institute of Medicine). 1997. *America's Vital Interest in Global Health: Protecting Our Republic, Enhancing our Economy, and Advancing our International Interests.* Washington, DC: National Academy Press.

———. 2009. *Beyond the HIPAA Privacy Rule: Enhancing Privacy, Improving Health through Research*. Washington, DC: National Academy Press.

Ioannidis, John P. A. 2013. "Informed Consent, Big Data, and the Oxymoron of Research That Is Not Research." *American Journal of Bioethics* 13(4): 40–42.

Jacka, Tamara. 2006. *Rural Women in Urban China: Gender, Migration, and Social Change*. Armonk, NY: M. E. Sharpe.

James, Erica C. 2008. "Haunting Ghosts: Madness, Gender, and *Ensekirite* in Haiti in the Democratic Era." In *Postcolonial Disorders*. Edited by M. D. Good, S. T. Hyde, S. Pinto, and B. J. Good, 132–156. Berkeley: University of California Press.

Janies, Daniel, Farhat Habib, Boyan Alexandrov, Andrew Hill, and Diego Pol. 2008. "Evolution of Genomes, Host Shifts and the Geographic Spread of SARS-CoV and Related Coronaviruses." *Cladistics* 24(2): 111–130.

Jasanoff, Sheila. 2004. *States of Knowledge*. New York: Routledge.

Jing, Jun. 2011. "From Commodity of Death to Gift of Life." In *Deep China: Remaking the Moral Person in a New China*, 78–105. Berkeley: University of California Press.

Kan, Biao, Ming Wang, Huaiqi Jing, Huifang Xu, Xiugao Jiang, Meiying Yan, et al. 2005. "Molecular Evolution Analysis and Geographic Investigation of Severe Acute Respiratory Syndrome Coronavirus-Like Virus in Palm Civets at an Animal Market and on Farms." *Journal of Virology* 79(18): 11892–11900.

Kass, Nancy E. 2001. "An Ethics Framework for Public Health." *American Journal of Public Health* 91(11): 1776–1782.

Kaufman, Joan A. 2006. "SARS and China's Health-Care Response: Better to Be Both Red and Expert!" In *SARS in China: Prelude to Pandemic?* Edited by Arthur Kleinman and J. Watson, 53–70. Stanford, CA: Stanford University Press.

———. 2008. "China's Health Care System and Avian Influenza Preparedness." *The Journal of Infectious Diseases* 2008(197): S7–13.

Kim, Jim Yong, Joyce V. Millen, Alec Irwin, and John Gershman, eds. 2002. *Dying for Growth: Global Inequality and the Health of the Poor*. Monroe, ME: Common Courage Press.

King, Ambrose Yeo-chi. 1991. "Kuan-shi and Network Building: A Sociological Interpretation." *Daedalus* 120(2): 63–84.

King, Meredith L. 2007. "Immigrants in the U.S. Healthcare System: Five Myths that Misinform the American Public." Retrieved on August 13, 2010, from www.americanprogress.org/issues/2007/06/immigrant_health_report.html.

King, Nicholas B. 2002. "Security, Disease, Commerce: Ideologies of Postcolonial Global Health." *Social Studies of Science* 32(5–6): 763–789.

Kipnis, Andrew B. 1997. *Producing Guanxi: Sentiment, Self, and Subculture in a North China Village*. Durham, NC: Duke University Press.

———. 2002. "Zouping Christianity as Gendered Critique? An Ethnography of Political Potentials." *Anthropology and Humanism* 27(1): 80–96.

———. 2010. *Governing Educational Desire: Culture, Politics and Schooling in China.* Chicago: University of Chicago Press.

Kleinman, Arthur. 1988. *The Illness Narratives: Suffering, Healing, and the Human Condition.* New York: Basic Books.

———. 1995. *Writing at the Margins: Discourse between Anthropology and Medicine.* Berkeley: University of California Press.

———. 1998. "Experience and Its Moral Modes: Culture, Human Conditions, and Disorder." *The Tanner Lectures on Human Values*, 357–420. Retrieved on August 13, 2010, from www.tannerlectures.utah.edu/lectures/atoz.html#k.

———. 2010. "Remaking the Moral Person in China: Implications for Health." *Lancet* 375(9720): 1074–1075.

Kleinman, Arthur, and James L. Watson, eds. 2006. *SARS in China: Prelude to Pandemic?* Stanford, CA: Stanford University Press.

Kleinman, Arthur, Yunxiang Yan, Jing Jun, Sing Lee, Everett Zhang, Pan Tianshu, Wu Fei, and Jinhua Guo. 2011. *Deep China: Remaking the Moral Person in a New China.* Berkeley: University of California Press.

Kleinman, Arthur M., Barry R. Bloom, Anthony Saich, Katherine A. Mason, and Felicity Aulino. 2008. "Introduction: Asian Flus in Ethnographic and Political Perspective: A Biosocial Approach." *Anthropology and Medicine* 15(1): 1–5.

Kohrman, Matthew. 2004. "Should I Quit? Tobacco, Fraught Identity, and the Risks of Governmentality in Urban China." *Urban Anthropology and Studies of Cultural Systems and World Economic Development* 33(2): 211–245.

———. 2005. *Bodies of Difference: Experiences of Disability and Institutional Advocacy in the Making of Modern China.* Berkeley: University of California Press.

Koplan, Jeffery P., T. Christopher Bond, Michael H. Merson, K. Srinath Reddy, Mario Henry Rodriguez, Nelson K. Sewankambo, and Judith N Wasserheit. 2009. "Towards a Common Definition of Global Health." *The Lancet* 373: 1993–1995.

Kuhn, Thomas. 1962. *The Structure of Scientific Revolutions.* Chicago: University of Chicago Press.

Kultgen, John. 1988. *Ethics and Professionalism.* Philadelphia: University of Pennsylvania Press.

Lakoff, Andrew, and Stephen J. Collier, eds. 2008. *Biosecurity Interventions: Global Health and Security in Question.* New York: Columbia University Press.

Lam, Kelvin K. F., and Janice M. Johnston. 2012. "Health Insurance and Healthcare Utilization for Shenzhen Residents: A Tale of Registrants and Migrants?" *BMC Public Health* 12: 868.

Larson, Eric B. 2013. "Building Trust in the Power of 'Big Data' Research to Serve the Public Good." *Journal of the American Medical Association* 309(23): 2443–2444.

Larson, Magali S. 1977. *The Rise of Professionalism: A Sociological Analysis*. Berkeley: University of California Press.

Latour, Bruno. 1993. *We Have Never Been Modern*. Translated by Catherine Porter. Cambridge, MA: Harvard University Press.

———. 1999. *Pandora's Hope: Essays on the Reality of Science Studies*. Cambridge, MA: Harvard University Press.

Latour, Bruno, and Steve Woolgar. 1979. *Laboratory Life: The Social Construction of Scientific Facts*. Beverley Hills, CA: Sage Publications.

Lau, Susanna K. P., Patrick C. Y. Woo, Kenneth S. M. Li, Yi Huang, Hoi-Wah Tsoi, et al. 2005. "Severe Acute Respiratory Syndrome Coronavirus-Like Virus in Chinese Horseshoe Bats." *Proceedings of the National Academy of Sciences* 102(39): 14040–14045.

Lee, Haiyan. 2014. *The Stranger and the Chinese Moral Imagination*. Stanford, CA: Stanford University Press.

Lee, Liming. 2004. "The Current State of Public Health in China." *Annual Review of Public Health* 25: 327–339.

Levi-Strauss, Claude. 1969 [1964]. *The Raw and the Cooked*. Translated by J. and D. Weightman. Chicago: University of Chicago Press.

Levinas, Emmanuel. 1988. "Useless Suffering." Translated by Richard Cohen. In *The Provocation of Levinas: Rethinking the Other*. Edited by Robert Bernasconi and David Wood, 156–167. New York: Routledge.

Lewis, Jane. 1991. "The Public's Health: Philosophy and Practice in Britain in the Twentieth Century." In *A History of Education in Public Health: Health That Mocks the Doctor's Rules*. Edited by E. Fee and R. M. Acheson, 195–229. New York: Oxford University Press.

Li Jianzhong and Deng Huihong. 2004. "Reflections on Tactics for Preventing and Treating Guangdong Infectious Atypical Pneumonia" [*Guangdong Chuanranxing Feidianxing Feiyan Fangzhi Celue de Sikao*]. *China Journal of Public Health Management* [*Zhongguo Gonggong Weisheng Guanli*] 20(4): 291–294.

Lieberthal, Kenneth. 1995. *Governing China: From Revolution through Reform*. New York: W. W. Norton.

Liu, J., H. Y. Yao, and E. Y. Liu. 2006. "Analysis of Factors Affecting the Epidemiology of Tuberculosis in China." *International Journal of Tuberculosis and Lung Disease* 9(4): 450–454.

Liu, Yuanli. 2004. "China's Public Health Care System: Facing the Challenges." *Bulletin of the World Health Organization* 82(7): 532–538.

Liu, Yuanli, and Joan Kaufman. 2006. "Controlling HIV/AIDS in China: Health System Challenges." In *AIDS and Social Policy in China*. Edited by Joan

Kaufman, Arthur Kleinman, and Tony Saich, 75–95. Cambridge, MA: Harvard Asia Center.

Lockerbie, Stacy, and D. Ann Herring. 2009. "Global Panic, Local Repercussions: Economic and Nutritional Effects of Bird Flu in Vietnam." In *Anthropology and Public Health: Bridging Differences in Culture and Society*, second edition. Edited by Robert A. Hahn and Marcia Claire Inhorn, 566–587. New York: Oxford University Press.

Lowe, Celia. 2006. *Wild Profusion: Biodiversity Conservation in an Indonesian Archipelago*. Princeton, NJ: Princeton University Press.

Lu, Xiaobo, and Elizabeth J. Perry. 1997. "Introduction: The Changing Chinese Workplace in Historical and Comparative Perspective." In *Danwei: The Changing Chinese Workplace in Historical and Comparative Perspective*. Edited by Xiaobo Lu and Elizabeth J. Perry, 1–20. New York: M. E. Sharpe.

Lu Yun and Li Liming. 2006. "Comparison of Our Country's CDC and Health Inspection System Functions and Current Public Health System Functions and Meanings" [*Woguo Jikong He Jiandu Tixi Zhineng Yu Xiandai Gonggong Weisheng Tixi Zhineng Neihan de Bijiao*]. *China Journal of Public Health Management* [*Zhongguo Gonggong Weisheng Guanli*] 22(5): 365–367.

———. 2007. "The Basic Functions and Meanings of Today's Public Health System" [*Xiandai Gonggong Weisheng Tixi de Jiben Zhineng Ji Qi Neihan*]. *China Journal of Public Health* [*Zhongguo Gonggong Weisheng*] 23(8): 1022–1024.

Luo Dezhi, Yang Jie, Luo Mengying, and Peng Hong. 2006. "Developmental, Conceptual, and Theoretical Views of Mass Participation in Public Health in Our Country" [*Woguo Gongxiong Canyu Gonggong Weisheng de Fazhan, Gainian Jiqi Lilun Jianshi*]. *Health Soft Science* [*Weisheng Ruankexue*] 20(4): 382–384.

Lurie, Nicole. 2009. "The Need for Science in the Practice of Public Health." *New England Journal of Medicine* 361(26): 2571–2572.

Ma, Chao, Lixin Hao, Yan Zhang, Qiru Su, Lance Rodewald, Zhijie An, Wenzhou Yu, Jing Ma, Ning Wen, Huiling Wang, Xiaofeng Liang, Huaqing Wang, Weizhong Yang, Li Li, and Huiming Luo. 2014. "Monitoring Progress towards the Elimination of Measles in China: An Analysis of Measles Surveillance Data." *Bulletin of the World Health Organization*. 2014(92): 340–347.

MacPhail, Theresa. 2014. *The Viral Network: A Pathology of the H1N1 Influenza Pandemic*. Ithaca, NY: Cornell University Press.

Magnier, Mark. 2014. "China's Migrant Workers Struggle for Pensions." *Wall Street Journal*, December 26.

Markel, Howard. 1997. *Quarantine! East European Jewish Immigrants and the New York City Epidemics of 1892*. Baltimore, MD: Johns Hopkins University Press.

Mason, Katherine A. 2010. "Becoming Modern after SARS: Battling H1N1 and the Politics of Backwardness in China's Pearl River Delta." Special Issue, "Epidemic Orders." *Behemoth: A Journal on Civilisation* 2010(3): 8–35.

———. 2013. "To Your Health! Toasting, Intoxication, and Gendered Critique among Banqueting Women." *The China Journal* 69: 108–133.

———. 2015. "H1N1 Is Not a Chinese Virus: The Racialization of People and Viruses in Post-SARS China." *Studies in Comparative International Development* 50(4): 500–518.

———. In press. "The Correct Secret: Discretion and Hypertransparency in Chinese Biosecurity." *Focaal: Journal of Global and Historical Anthropology.*

Mausezahl, Daniel, Feng Cheng, Shaoqing Q. Zhang, and Marcel Tanner. 1996. "Hepatitis A in a Chinese Urban Population: The Spectrum of Social and Behavioural Risk Factors." *International Journal of Epidemiology* 25(6): 1271–1275.

McKeown, Thomas, and Robert G. Brown. 1955. "Medical Evidence Related to English Population Changes in the Eighteenth Century." *Population Studies* 9: 119–141.

McNeil, Donald G. Jr. 2014. "Using a Tactic Unseen in a Century, Countries Cordon off Ebola-Racked Areas." *New York Times*, August 13, A10.

Mertha, Andrew C. 2005. *The Politics of Piracy: Intellectual Property in Contemporary China*. Ithaca, NY: Cornell University Press.

Metzl, Jonathan M. 2009. "China's Ill-Considered Response to the H1N1 Virus." *Los Angeles Times*, July 12. Retrieved on July 13, 2009, from http://articles.latimes.com/2009/jul/12/opinion/oe-metzl12.

Molina, Natalia. 2006. *Fit to be Citizens? Public Health and Race in Los Angeles, 1879–1939*. Berkeley: University of California Press.

Montoya, Michael J. 2007. "Bioethnic Conscription: Genes, Race, and Mexicana/o Ethnicity in Diabetes Research." *Cultural Anthropology* 22(1): 94–128.

Moran-Thomas, Amy. 2013. "A Salvage Ethnography of the Guinea Worm: Witchcraft, Oracles, and Magic in a Disease Eradication Program." In *When People Come First: Critical Studies in Global Health*. Edited by Joao Biehl and Adriana Petryna, 207–242. Princeton, NJ: Princeton University Press.

Mou Jin, Jinquan Cheng, Dan Zhang, Hanping Jiang, Liangqiang Lin, and Sian M Griffiths. 2009. "Health Care Utilisation among Shenzhen Migrant Workers: Does Being Insured Make a Difference?" *BMC Health Services Research* 9: 214–222.

Mou Jin, Sian M. Griffiths, Hildy Fong, and Martin G. Dawes. 2013. "Health of China's Rural to Urban Migrants and Their Families: A Review of Literature From 2000 to 2012." *British Medical Bulletin* 106: 19–43.

Murphy, Priscilla. 2001. "Affiliation Bias and Expert Disagreement in Framing the Nicotine Addiction Debate." *Science, Technology and Human Values* 26(3): 278–299.

Murphy, Rachel. 2002. *How Migrant Labor Is Changing Rural China*. Cambridge, UK: Cambridge University Press.

Nancy, Jean-Luc. 1991. *The Inoperative Community*. Minneapolis: University of Minnesota Press.

NHPHSQE (National Health Professional Health Skills Qualification Exam) Expert Committee [Quanguo Weisheng Zhuanye Jishu Zige Kaoshi Zhuanjia Weiyuanhui]. 2009. *National Health Professional Health Skills Qualification Exam Guide [Quanguo Weishengg Zhuanye Jishu Zige Kaoshi Zhidao]*. Beijing: People's Health Publishing House [Renmin Weisheng Chubanshe].

Navarro, Vicente. 1984. "A Critique of the Ideological and Political Positions of the Willy Brandt Report and the WHO Alma Ata Declaration." *Social Science and Medicine* 18(6): 467–474.

Newendorp, Nicole D. 2008. *Uneasy Reunions: Immigration, Citizenship, and Family Life in Post-1997 Hong Kong*. Stanford, CA: Stanford University Press.

Ngai, Pun. 2005. *Made in China: Women Factory Workers in a Global Workplace*. Durham, NC: Duke University Press.

Nguyen, Vinh-Kim. 2010. *The Republic of Therapy: Triage and Sovereignty in West Africa's Time of AIDS*. Durham, NC: Duke University Press.

Nichter, Mark. 2008. *Global Health: Why Cultural Perceptions, Social Representations, and Biopolitics Matter*. Tucson, AZ: University of Arizona Press.

Nie, Jing Bao. 2001. "Challenges of Japanese Doctors' Human Experimentation in China for East-Asian and Chinese Bioethics." *Eubios Journal of Asian and International Bioethics* 11: 3–7.

Nie, Jing Bao, Nanyan Guo, Mark Selden, and Arthur Kleinman. 2010. *Japan's Wartime Medical Atrocities: Comparative Inquiries in Science, History and Ethics*. New York: Routledge.

Oakley, Justin, and Dean Cocking. 2001. *Virtue Ethics and Professional Roles*. New York: Cambridge University Press.

O'Donnell, Mary Ann. 2001. "Becoming Hong Kong, Razing Bao'an, Preserving Xin'An: An Ethnographic Account of Urbanization in the Shenzhen Special Economic Zone." *Cultural Studies* 15(3–4): 419–443.

Oksenberg, Michel C. 1974. "Chinese Politics and the Public Health Issue." In *Medicine and Society in China*, edited by J. Z. Bowers and E. F. Purcell, 128–160. New York: Josiah Macy Jr. Foundation.

Ong, Aihwa. 1999. *Flexible Citizenship: The Cultural Logics of Transnationality*. Durham, NC: Duke University Press.

———. 2006. *Neoliberalism as Exception: Mutations in Citizenship and Sovereignty*. Durham, NC: Duke University Press.

Ong, Aihwa, and Li Zhang. 2008. "Introduction: Privatizing China: Powers of the Self, Socialism from Afar." In *Privatizing China: Socialism from Afar*. Edited by Aihwa Ong and Li Zhang, 1–20. Berkeley: University of California Press.

Onishi, Norimitsu. 2014. "Clashes Erupt as Liberia Sets an Ebola Quarantine." *New York Times*, August 21, A1.

Osburg, John. 2013. *Anxious Wealth: Money and Morality among China's New Rich.* Stanford, CA: Stanford University Press.

Otte, Joachim. 2006. "The Hen Which Lays the Golden Eggs: Why Backyard Poultry Are So Popular." *Pro-Poor Livestock Policy Initiative.* Retrieved on March 18, 2007, from www.fao.org/ag/AGAInfo/projects/en/pplpi/docarc/featureo1_backyardpoultry.pdf.

Oxfeld, Ellen. 2010. *Drink Water but Remember the Source: Moral Discourse in a Chinese Village.* Berkeley: University of California Press.

Peckham, Stephen, and Alison Hann, eds. 2009. *Public Health Ethics and Practice.* Portland, OR: The Policy Press.

Peng, Jing, Sheng Nian Zhang, Wei Lu, and Andrew T. L. Chen. 2003. "Public Health in China: The Shanghai CDC Perspective." *American Journal of Public Health* 93(12): 1991–1993.

PRC (People's Republic of China) Ministry of Health. 2006. "Human Highly Pathogenic Avian Influenza Emergency Plan" [*Renganran Gaozhi Bingxing Qinliugan Yingji Yu'an*]. Retrieved on March 18, 2007, from www.moh.gov.cn/open/uploadfile/20067129433061262.doc.

———. 2007a. "Clearly Examine Unclear Cases, Effective Preparation Prevents SARS from Returning" [*Mingcha Anfang Zuo Zu Zhunbei Gongzuo, Youxiao Fangzhi Feidian Zaici Fasheng*]. Retrieved on April 7, 2007, from www.gov.cn/zxft/ft11/content_573638.hSZ.

———. 2007b. "Spread Health Knowledge, Decrease the Rate of Occurrence of Public Health Emergencies" [*Guangfan Puji Weisheng Zhishi, Jiangdi Tufa Gonggong Weisheng Shijian de Fashenglu*]. Retrieved on April 7, 2007, from www.gov.cn/zxft/ft11/content_573618.hSZ.

———. 2009a. "Implementation Plan for Deepening of Health Care System Reform" [*2009–2011 Shenhua Yiliao Weisheng Tizhi Gaige Shishi Fang'an*]. Retrieved on April 6, 2010, from www.gov.cn/zwgk/2009-04/07/content_1279256.hSZ.

———. 2009b. "Ministry of Health Ethics Investigations for Biomedical Research Involving Human Subjects" [*Weisheng Bu Sheji Renti de Shengwu Yixue Lunli Shencha Banfa*]. Retrieved on November 23, 2010, from www.chinaids.org.cn/worknet/irb/doc/t6_cn.doc.

People's Republic of China Ministry of Health, China Centers for Disease Control and Prevention, United States Department of Health and Human Services, and United States Centers for Disease Control and Prevention. 2007. Newsletter. "China–U.S. Collaborative Program on Emerging and Re-Emerging Infectious Diseases China–US CDC Component 1," 1–8.

Petryna, Adriana. 2002. *Life Exposed: Biological Citizens after Chernobyl.* Princeton, NJ: Princeton University Press.

———. 2005. "Ethical Variability: Drug Development and the Globalization of Clinical Trials." *American Ethnologist* 32(2): 183–197.

————. 2009. *When Experiments Travel: Clinical Trials and the Global Search for Human Subjects.* Princeton, NJ: Princeton University Press.

Pollock, Anne. 2012. *Medicating Race: Heart Disease and Durable Preoccupations with Difference.* Durham, NC: Duke University Press.

Poo, Mu-Ming. 2004. "Cultural Reflections." *Nature* 428: 204–205.

Porter, Dorothy. 1991. "Stratification and Its Discontents: Professionalization and Conflict in the British Public Health Service." In *A History of Education in Public Health: Health That Mocks the Doctor's Rules.* Edited by Elizabeth Fee and Roy M. Acheson, 83–113. New York: Oxford University Press.

Raffoul, Francois. 2010. *The Origins of Responsibility.* Bloomington: Indiana University Press.

Rajan, Kaushik S. 2006. *Biocapital: The Constitution of Postgenomic Life.* Durham, NC: Duke University Press.

Reddy, Deepa S. 2007. "Good Gifts for the Common Good: Blood and Bioethics in the Market of Genetic Research." *Cultural Anthropology* 22(3): 429–472.

Reuters. 2010. "Experts Open Review of WHO Response to Swine Flu." *Reuters,* April 12.

Rogaski, Ruth. 2004. *Hygienic Modernity: Meanings of Health and Disease in Treaty-Port China.* Berkeley: University of California Press.

Rose, Nikolas. 2006. *The Politics of Life Itself: Biomedicine, Power, and Subjectivity in the Twenty-First Century.* Princeton, NJ: Princeton University Press.

Rosen, George. 1993 [1958]. *A History of Public Health,* expanded edition. Baltimore, MD: Johns Hopkins University Press.

Rosenberg, Charles E. 1987 [1962]. *The Cholera Years: The United States in 1832, 1849, and 1866,* second edition. Chicago: University of Chicago Press.

Rosenkrantz, Barbara G. 1972. *Public Health and the State: Changing Views in Massachusetts 1842–1936.* Cambridge, MA: Harvard University Press.

————. 1974. "Cart before Horse: Theory, Practice and Professional Image in American Public Health, 1870–1920." *Journal of the History of Medicine* 29(1): 55–73.

Rosenthal, Marilynn M. 1987. *Health Care in the People's Republic of China: Moving Toward Modernization.* Boulder, CO: Westview Press.

Rothman, David. 2000. "The Shame of Medical Research." *New York Review of Books* XLV: 60–64.

Rothstein, Mark D. 2015. "From SARS to Ebola: Legal and Ethical Considerations for Modern Quarantine." *Indiana Health Law Review* 12(1).

Rothstein, Mark D., and Abigail B. Shoben. 2013. "Does Consent Bias Research?" *American Journal of Bioethics* 13(4): 27–37.

Saich, Tony. 2006. "Is SARS China's Chernobyl or Much Ado about Nothing?" In *SARS in China: Prelude to Pandemic?* Edited by Arthur Kleinman and James Watson, 71–104. Stanford, CA: Stanford University Press.

Sankar, Pamela. 2004. "Communication and Miscommunication in Informed Consent to Research." *Medical Anthropology Quarterly* 18(4): 429–444.

Sassen, Saskia. 2006. *Territory, Authority, Rights: From Medieval to Global Assemblages.* Princeton, NJ: Princeton University Press.

Schutz, Alfred. 1967 [1932]. *The Phenomenology of the Social World.* Evanston, IL: Northwestern University Press.

Shah, Nayan. 2001. *Contagious Divides: Epidemics and Race in San Francisco's Chinatown.* Berkeley: University of California Press.

Shapin, Steven. 1994. *A Social History of Truth: Civility and Science in Seventeenth-Century England.* Chicago: University of Chicago Press.

———. 1998. "Placing the View from Nowhere: Historical and Sociological Problems in the Location of Science." *Transactions of the Institute of British Geographers, NS* 23: 5–12.

Shortridge, Kennedy F. 2003. "Severe Acute Respiratory Syndrome and Influenza: Virus Incursions from Southern China." *American Journal of Respiratory Critical Care Medicine* 168: 1416–1420.

Sidel, Ruth, and Victor W. Sidel. 1977. "Health Care Services." *Social Scientist* 5(10): 112–130.

Sidel, Victor W., and Ruth Sidel. 1982. *The Health of China.* Boston: Beacon Press.

Sigley, Gary. 2006. "Chinese Governmentalities: Government, Governance and the Socialist Market Economy." *Economy and Society* 35(4): 487–508.

Simon, Denis F., and Merle Goldman, eds. 1989. *Science and Technology in Post-Mao China.* Cambridge, MA: The Council on East Asian Studies, Harvard University.

Singer, Merrill. 2009. "Pathogens Gone Wild? Medical Anthropology and the 'Swine Flu' Pandemic." *Medical Anthropology* 28(3): 199–206.

Siu, Helen F. 2007. "Grounding Displacement: Uncivil Urban Spaces in Post-Reform South China." *American Anthropologist* 34(2): 329–350.

Sleigh, A., S. Jackson, X. Li, and K. Huang. 1998. "Eradication of Schistosomiasis in Guangxi, China. Part 2: Political Economy, Management Strategy and Costs, 1953–92." *Bulletin of the World Health Organization* 76(5): 497–508.

Smith, Mark, George Halvorson, and Gary Kaplan. 2012. "What's Needed Is a Health Care System That Learns: Recommendations from an IOM Report." *Journal of the American Medical Association* 308(16): 1637–1638.

Solinger, Dorothy J. 1999. *Contesting Citizenship in Urban China: Peasant Migrants, the State, and the Logic of the Market.* Berkeley: University of California Press.

Spencer, Jonathan. 2001. "Ethnography after Postmodernism." In *Handbook of Ethnography.* Edited by P. Atkinson et al., 443–452. London: Sage.

Starr, Paul. 1982. *The Social Transformation of American Medicine.* New York: Basic Books.

Steele, Liza G., and Scott M. Lynch. 2012. "The Pursuit of Happiness in China: Individualism, Collectivism, and Subjective Well-Being During China's Economic and Social Transformation." *Social Indicators Research* 114(2): 441–451.

Stevenson, Lisa. 2012. "The Psychic Life of Biopolitics: Survival, Cooperation, and Inuit Community." *American Ethnologist* 39(3): 592–613.

Stolberg, S. G., and O. Robinson. 2009. "Swine Flu Diary: Caught in a Beijing Dragnet." *New York Times*, July 28, D1.

Strathern, Marilyn, ed. 2000a. *Audit Cultures: Anthropological Studies in Accountability, Ethics and the Academy.* New York: Routledge.

———. 2000b. "The Tyranny of Transparency." *British Educational Research Journal* 26(4): 309–321.

Sun Wenjie 2004. "Research on the Application of the Principle of Informed Consent during Field Investigations" [*Xianchang Diaochazhong Zhiqing Tongyi Yuanze de Yingyong Yanjiu*]. *China Medical Ethics* [*Zhongguo Yixue Lunlixue*] 17(5): 13–17.

Tang, Shenglan, Qingyue Meng, Lincoln Chen, Henk Bekedam, Tim Evans, and Margaret Whitehead. 2008. "Tackling the Challenges to Health Equity in China." *The Lancet* 372(9648): 25–31.

Ticktin, Miriam. 2006. "Where Ethics and Politics Meet: The Violence of Humanitarianism in France." *American Ethnologist* 33(1): 33–49.

Tiezzi, Shannon. 2014. "China Sends Aid, Medical Teams to Fight Ebola Outbreak." *The Diplomat*, August 12.

Tomba, Luigi. 2014. *The Government Next Door: Neighborhood Politics in Urban China.* Ithaca, NY: Cornell University Press.

Tomes, Nancy. 1998. *The Gospel of Germs: Men, Women, and the Microbe in American Life.* Cambridge, MA: Harvard University Press.

Tu Wei-ming. 1979. *Humanity and Self-Cultivation: Essays in Confucian Thought.* Berkeley, CA: Asian Humanities Press.

———. 1985. *Confucian Thought: Selfhood as Creative Transformation.* Albany: State University of New York Press.

Turnock, Bernard J. 2012. *Essentials of Public Health*, second edition. Sudbury, MA: Jones and Bartlett Learning.

UNDP (United Nations Development Programme). December 2014. *Issue Brief: The Ebola Virus Outbreak and China's Response.* No. 6. Beijing: Author.

U.S. CDC (United States Centers for Disease Control and Prevention). 2001. *Protecting the Nation's Health in an Era of Globalization: CDC's Global Infectious Disease Strategy.* Atlanta, GA: U.S. Department of Health and Human Services, Public Health Service.

———. 2009. "CHINA Field Epidemiology Training Program Fact Sheet." Electronic Document, retrieved on March 10, 2011, from www.cdc.gov/globalhealth/FETP/pdf/China_factsheet.pdf.

U.S. Department of Health and Human Services. 2005. "HHS Pandemic Influenza Plan." Retrieved on June 3, 2010, from www.hhs.gov/pandemicflu/plan/.

U.S. Homeland Security Council. 2006. "National Strategy for Pandemic Influenza: Implementation Plan." Retrieved on June 2, 2010, from http://georgewbushwhitehouse.archives.gov/homeland/pandemic-influenza-implementation.html.

Uretsky, Elanah. 2008. "Mobile Men with Money: The Socio-Cultural and Politico-Economic Context of 'High-Risk' Behavior among Wealthy Businessmen and Government Officials in Urban China," *Culture, Health and Sexuality* 10(8): 801–814.

Wagner, John R. 2012. "Water and the Commons Imaginary." *Current Anthropology* 53(5): 617–641.

Wald, Priscilla. 2008. *Contagious: Cultures, Carriers, and the Outbreak Narratives.* Durham, NC: Duke University Press.

Waldby, Catherine, and Robert Mitchell. 2006. *Tissue Economies: Gifts, Commodities, and Bio-Value in Late Capitalism.* Durham, NC: Duke University Press.

Walsh, Bryan. 2009. "CDC's Dr. Richard Besser on Swine Flu and Katrina." *Time Magazine*, May 5. Retrieved on January 16, 2010, from www.time.com/time/health/article/0,8599,1895820,00.hSZl.

Wang, Longde, Jianjun Liu, and Daniel P. Chin. 2007. "Progressing Tuberculosis Control and the Evolving Public Health System in China." *The Lancet* 369: 691–696.

Wang Qing. 2003. "Investigation and Analysis of Patient Informed Consent" [*Guanyu Bingren Zhiqing Tongyi de Diaocha yu Fenxi*]. *China Public Health* [*Zhongguo Gonggong Weisheng*] 19(1).

Warren, Kenneth. 1988. "'Farewell to the Plague Spirit': Chairman Mao's Crusade against Schistosomiasis." In *Science and Medicine in Twentieth-Century China: Research and Education*, edited by John Z. Bowers, William J. Hess, and Nathan Sivin, 123–140. Ann Arbor: Center for Chinese Studies, University of Michigan.

Watson, James L. 2004. "Presidential Address: Virtual Kinship, Real Estate, and Diaspora Formation—The Man Lineage Revisited." *The Journal of Asian Studies* 63(4): 893–910.

Weber, Max. 1978. *Economy and Society*, Vol. 2. Translated by G. Roth and C. Wittich. Berkeley: University of California Press.

———. 2002. *The Protestant Ethic and the Spirit of Capitalism.* Translated by T. Parsons. New York: Routledge.

Weed, Douglas L., and Robert E. McKeown. 1993. "Science and Social Responsibility in Public Health." *Environmental Health Perspectives* 111(14): 1804–1808.

———. 1998. "Epidemiology and Virtue Ethics." *International Journal of Epidemiology* 27: 343–349.

Weiser, Benjamin, and J. David Goodman. 2014. "The Flu, TB, and Now Ebola: A Rare Legal Remedy Returns." *New York Times*, Oct. 26.

Wendland, Claire L. 2012. "Moral Maps and Medical Imaginaries: Clinical Tourism at Malawi's College of Medicine." *American Anthropologist* 11(1): 108–122.

Whyte, Susan Reynolds, Michael A. Whyte, Lotte Meinert, and Jenipher Twebaze. 2013. "Therapeutic Clientship: Belonging in Uganda's Projectified Landscape of AIDS Care." In *When People Come First: Critical Studies in Global Health*. Princeton, NJ: Princeton University Press.

Willen, Sarah S. 2007. "Toward a Critical Phenomenology of 'Illegality': State Power, Criminalization, and Abjectivity among Undocumented Migrant Workers in Tel Aviv, Israel." *International Migration* 45(3): 8–38.

Wong, Edward. 2009. "China's Tough Measures Appear to Be Effective." *New York Times*, November 12, A3.

WHO (World Health Organization). 2003. "Consensus Document on the Epidemiology of Severe Acute Respiratory Syndrome (SARS)." Geneva: World Health Organization, Department of Communicable Disease Surveillance and Response.

———. 2004. "Avian Influenza A(H5) in Rural Areas in Asia: Food Safety Considerations." Retrieved on March 17, 2007, from www.who.int/foodsafety/micro/avian2/en/.

———. 2005a. "Revision of the International Health Regulations." Retrieved on March 26, 2007, from www.who.int/csr/ihr/IHRWHA58_3-en.pdf.

———. 2005b. "WHO Global Influenza Preparedness Plan: The Role of WHO and Recommendations for National Measures Before and During Pandemics." Retrieved on March 13, 2007, from www.who.int/csr/resources/publications/influenza/GIP_2005_5Eweb.pdf.

———. 2007. "Ethical Considerations in Developing a Public Health Response to Pandemic Influenza." Retrieved on June 3, 2010, from www.who.int/csr/resources/publications/WHO_CDS_EPR_GIP_2007_2/en/index.hSZl.

———. 2009. "Pandemic Influenza Preparedness and Response: A WHO Guidance Document." Retrieved on June 3, 2010, from www.who.int/csr/disease/influenza/pipguidance2009/en/index.hSZl.

Wynia, Matthew K. 2007. "Ethics and Public Health Emergencies: Restrictions on Liberties." *American Journal of Bioethics* 7(2): 1–5.

Xiao Aishu. 2005. "Discussion of Mao Zedong's Historical Contribution to Our Country's Hygiene and Epidemic Prevention Undertaking" [*Lun Mao Zedong Dui Wo Guo Weisheng Fangyi shiye de Lishixing Gongxian*]. *Journal of Jining Teacher's College* [*Jining Shifan Zhuanke Xuexiao Xuebao*] 25(5): 17–22.

Xinhua. 2009. "WHO: No Fixed Prescription for Vigilance, Isolation/Quarantine Is an Established Principle." [*ShiWei: Fangfan Wu Guding Chufang, Geli Shi Jiding Yuanze*] *Southern Weekend* [*Nanfang Dushi Bao*] May 6, A06.

Yan Hairong. 2008. *New Masters, New Servants: Migration, Development, and Women Workers in China*. Durham, NC: Duke University Press.

Yan Yunxiang. 1996. *The Flow of Gifts: Reciprocity and Social Networks in a Chinese Village*. Stanford, CA: Stanford University Press.

———. 2003. *Private Life under Socialism: Love, Intimacy, and Family Change in a Chinese Village 1949–1999*. Stanford, CA: Stanford University Press

———. 2009. *The Individualization of Chinese Society*. New York: Berg.

Yang, Gonghuan, Lingzhi Kong, Wenhua Zhao, Xia Wan, Yi Zhai, Lincoln C. Chen, and Jeffrey P. Koplan. 2008. "Emergence of Chronic Non-Communicable Diseases in China." *The Lancet* 372: 1697–1705.

Yang, Mayfair M. 1994. *Gifts, Favors, and Banquets: The Art of Social Relationships in China*. Ithaca, NY: Cornell University Press.

Yao Lin and Liu Miaomiao. 2006. "Building a Protective Screen for the Health of the Common People: A Record of My District's Construction of Public Health Undertaking" [*Goujian Baixing Jiankang de Pingzhang: Wo Qu Gonggong Weisheng Shiye Jianshe Jishi*]. *Guangxi Daily* [*Guangxi Ribao*], December 9.

Yao, Xinzhong. 2000. *An Introduction to Confucianism*. Cambridge, UK: Cambridge University Press.

Yu Dongbao, Lenore Manderson, Liping Yuan, Wangyuan Wei, Hongbin He, and Yan Chen 2001. Is Equity Being Sacrificed? Willingness and Ability to Pay for Schistosomiasis Control in China. *Health Policy and Planning* 16(3): 292–301.

Zaidi, S.Akbar. 1999. "NGO Failure and the Need to Bring Back the State." *Journal of International Development* 11(2): 259.

Zhan, Mei. 2005. "Civet Cats, Fried Grasshoppers, and David Beckham's Pajamas: Unruly Bodies after SARS." *American Anthropologist* 107(1): 31–42.

Zhang, Jian, Yu Jing-Jin, Zhang Rong-Zhen, Zhang Xing-Lu, Zhou Jun, Jessie S. Wing, Alan Schnur, and Wang Ke-An. 1998. "Costs of Polio Immunization Days in China: Implications for Mass Immunization Campaign Strategies." *International Journal of Health Planning and Management* 13(1998): 5–25.

Zhang Lei, Eric Pui Fung Chow, Jun Zhang, Jun Jing, and David P. Wilson. 2012. "Describing the Chinese HIV Surveillance System and the Influences of Political Structures and Social Stigma." *The Open AIDS Journal* 6(Suppl 1: M14): 163–168.

Zhang, Li. 2001. *Strangers in the City: Reconfigurations of Space, Power, and Social Networks within China's Floating Population*. Stanford, CA: Stanford University Press.

———. 2010. *In Search of Paradise: Middle-Class Living in a Chinese Metropolis*. Ithaca, NY: Cornell University Press.

Zhang Yade, Jiang Meishu, Wu Yongsheng, Wu Xiaomin, Liu Dongming, Chi Xiumei, and Liu Ying. 2008. "Discussion of Existing Problems and Perfecting the Building of a Health Emergency Protocol Database in Shenzhen City"

[*Shenzhen Shi Weisheng Yingji Yu'anku Jianshe Cunzai de Wenti Yu Wanshan Chuangxin Tantao*]. *China Journal of Tropical Medicine* [*Zhongguo Redai Yixue*] 8(1): 121–124.

Zhong, Yang. 2003. *Local Government and Politics in China: Challenges from Below.* Armonk, NY: M. E. Sharpe.

Zhuang Pinghui. 2014. "Measles Makes a Comeback in China as Vaccination Falters among Migrant Workers." *South China Morning Post,* July 7.

Index

Tianmai: AES in, 10, 12; Bureau of
Health (BOH)/Health and Family
Planning Commission, 18, 30, 72, 73,
74, 75, 87, 94, 95, 107, 118, 154, 186,
213nn19,20; Center for Chronic Disease Prevention and Control (CCDC),
30; cuisine, 4–5; economic conditions,
21; Food and Drug Administration
(TM FDA), 30; Great Migrant Study
in, 117–29, 130, 131, 137, 138, 201; vs.
Guangzhou, 29, 30, 37, 116, 221n2;
Health Education Research Center,
30; Health Inspection Institute, 30;
and Hong Kong border, 4, 5–7, 28, 29,
150, 151, 152, 153–54; immigrants in,
4, 36, 37–52; Mental Health Center,
30; modernization of, 147; Occupational Health Institute, 30, 217n8;
population, 4, 211n4, 214n2; Quarantine Inspection and Control Bureau,
151, 153–54, 170; Tianmai dream,
37–38; villages in, 45–47
Tianmai Center for Disease Control
and Prevention (TM CDC), 4, 10, 20,
31–32, 217n9, 218n19; Department of
HIV/AIDS Prevention and Control,
71, 185–200, 201, 215n13, 216n18,
221nn3,4; departments of, 29–30,
213n24; director (*zhuren*), 25, 29, 31,
48, 87–88, 109, 110, 125, 151, 166–67,
169–70, 186; during H1N1 influenza
pandemic of 2009, 36, 143–46, 149–61;
promotional videos, 64; relations with
district-level CDCs, 46–47, 72–73,
75–77; relations with street-level
CDCs, 46–47, 72–73; sanitation inspections by, 82–84, 85; during SARS
outbreak, 2, 13–14; during Sichuan
earthquake, 14–16, 186; as work unit
(*danwei*), 18, 47–49, 50, 74, 87–91, 109,
110, 140, 213n18, 215n11. *See also* public health professionals; public health
research
Tibet, 55
Tomba, Luigi, 18, 25, 49, 212n10,
215nn9,11, 216n5
Traditional Chinese Medicine (TCM),
154, 160
trust: personal trust, 197; professionalized trust, 27, 69, 92, 93, 99–102, 103,

104–5, 126–27, 129, 158–59, 178, 196,
197; social trust/mistrust, 27–28, 35,
49, 85–86, 102, 103–4, 130–31, 133,
137, 139, 196–99, 200
truth, 77, 96–99, 101, 102, 171
Tu Wei-ming, 79, 197, 219n6
Tu Youyou, 112
tuberculosis, 10, 58–59, 75

Uganda, 219n4
Ukraine, 42
unemployment insurance, 39
United Kingdom: HIV blood-screening
program in, 136–37, 138; public health
vs. medicine in, 16–17
United Nations Programme on HIV
and AIDS (UNAIDS), 31, 101
United States: biomedical research ethics in, 116, 138; CDC, 10, 12, 31, 34,
85, 141, 146, 149, 151, 158, 160, 161,
162–63, 173, 186, 212n12; Department
of Health and Human Services, 161,
162, 163; Ebola in, 221n4; fabrication
of data in, 125; H1N1 in, 147–48, 149,
154, 159, 161–64, 165, 169, 173, 175,
178; Homeland Security Council, 161,
162; immigrants in, 214n5, 215n14;
informed consent in, 128–29, 130, 133,
138; public health ethics in, 136, 138,
183; public health institutions in, 141;
public health profession in, 213n17;
public health vs. medicine in, 16–17;
Tuskegee study, 139

vaccination, 14, 70, 97; for H1N1 influenza, 163; mass campaigns under Mao,
8, 25, 43; for measles, 42, 46, 74–77,
98–99
venereal disease, 8, 101–2
Venezuela, 20

Wald, Priscilla, 146, 147
Wang, Longde, 9, 11
Wang, Lyla, 100–102
Watson, James L., 6, 33, 62
wealthy population (*fuyou renkou*), 55
Weber, Max, 24, 69, 89
Weed, Douglas L., 132, 135
Wen Jiabao, 71, 186, 216n1
wenjian (official document), 74